Practical Record Book
for
General Nursing and Midwifery

Name of the Student: ____

Name of the Institution: ____

Practical Record Book
for
General Nursing and Midwifery

As per the INC Syllabus

SN Nanjunde Gowda MSc(N) PhD

Professor and *Former* Principal
Anil Baghi College of Nursing
Ferozepur, Punjab, India

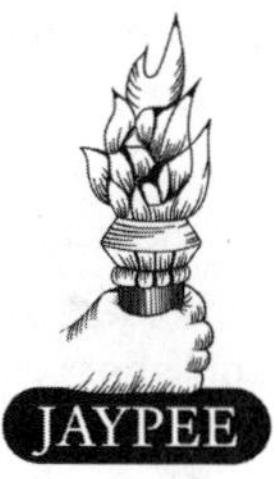

JAYPEE BROTHERS MEDICAL PUBLISHERS
The Health Sciences Publisher
New Delhi | London

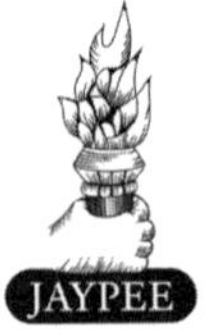 **Jaypee Brothers Medical Publishers (P) Ltd**

Headquarters

Jaypee Brothers Medical Publishers (P) Ltd
EMCA House
23/23-B, Ansari Road, Daryaganj
New Delhi - 110 002, India
Landline: +91-11-23272143, +91-11-23272703
+91-11-23282021, +91-11-23245672
Email: jaypee@jaypeebrothers.com

Corporate Office

Jaypee Brothers Medical Publishers (P) Ltd
4838/24, Ansari Road, Daryaganj
New Delhi 110 002, India
Phone: +91-11-43574357
Fax: +91-11-43574314
Email: jaypee@jaypeebrothers.com

Website: www.jaypeebrothers.com

Website: www.jaypeedigital.com

Overseas Office

J.P. Medical Ltd
83 Victoria Street, London
SW1H 0HW (UK)
Phone: +44 20 3170 8910
Fax: +44 (0)20 3008 6180
Email: info@jpmedpub.com

Practical Record Book for General Nursing and Midwifery

First Edition: **2024**

ISBN: 978-93-5696-896-7

Printed at: Sterling Graphics Pvt. Ltd. India.

Preface

Education technology refers to the development of various methods of educational technological inventions. These advances come from the interaction of changing concepts with changing techniques leading to new ways of performing educational activities.

The basics of nursing education depend on theory, clinical exposure and quality of nursing education. A nursing educator has great responsibilities to develop psychomotor and technical skills in the learner. If the theory and clinical experience is systematically planned, organized and adheres to the criteria, we can expect to impart nursing skills in the learner. A nursing educational institute plays a vital role in providing clinical learning experience according to prescribed educational requirements.

It is the responsibility of a clinical teacher to discuss a student's progress and clinical performance on a continuous basis. Strengths and weaknesses of the students should be identified, documented, and reported. A student's signature on each subject only indicates that she/he has practiced.

This practical record book is prepared according to the INC syllabus for General Nursing and Midwifery course.

SN Nanjunde Gowda

Acknowledgments

Preparation of this *Practical Record Book for General Nursing and Midwifery* resulted from the support of my students and colleagues. As an author, I acknowledge their support and professionalism. I am very proud to be associated with such fine individuals. My special thanks go to nursing teachers and students who supported me.

My sincere thought is that if the nursing teacher, students, and other healthcare providers personally apply the scientific principles described in this book, I will get immense satisfaction. I sincerely welcome constructive criticism from users that will help me to enrich my knowledge to contribute more to the profession.

I am very grateful to the whole team of M/s Jaypee Brothers Medical Publishers (P) Ltd, New Delhi, India, especially Shri Jitendar P Vij (Group Chairman), Mr Ankit Vij (Managing Director), Mr MS Mani (Group President), Dr Madhu Choudhary (Director–Educational Publishing), Ms Pooja Bhandari [Director-Production (Books and Journals)], Ms Sunita Katla (Executive Assistant to Group Chairman and Publishing Manager), Mr Ajay Kumar Sharma [Deputy General Manager (Books and Journals)], Ms Teresa Lamniang (Development Editor–Nursing), Mr Rajesh Sharma (Production Coordinator), Ms Seema Dogra (Cover Visualizer), Ms Neha Verma (Graphic Designer), Ms Geeta Barik (Proofreader), Mr Kapil Dev Sharma (Typesetter), and their team members, for all their support to work in this project and make it a success.

Above all, I am thankful to Almighty God for bestowing his bountiful grace for completion of this book.

SN Nanjunde Gowda

Contents

CLINICAL PRACTICE RECORD
STUDENT PROFILE

PHOTO

Name of the Student: ____

Date of Birth: ____

Name of the Father: ____

Name of the Mother: ____

Role Number/Registration Number: ____

Session: ____

Name of the Institute: ____

Address of Institute: ____

____

____

Signature of Student   Signature of Subject In-charge

Signature of HOD   Signature of Principal

A NURSES PRAYER

As I care for my patients today be there with me,
Oh Lord, I pray.
Make my word kind,
it means so much.
And in my hands, place your healing touch.
Let your love shine through in all that I do.
So those who are in need may hear you,
feel you and see you in me.

TEACHING IN CLINICAL SETTING

■ INTRODUCTION

Clinical experiences refer to the activities where students are exposed in attending health care of the clients, in which student applies knowledge and develops skills. Clinical learning experience requires a sound understanding of the curriculum, the learner and the learning environment and expertise of the teacher.

Understanding the Students

Faculty must have full knowledge and understanding of each student. Students differ in their level of learning and preferences for learning opportunities. Clinical teacher make assessment about student whether student possess the psychomotor and decision-making skill needed for providing care. Clinical faculty must evaluate the student in cognitive, psychomotor and affective domains. The evaluation must be on going and assist the student in learning and give constructive and timely feedback which promote achievement of goal.

Characteristics of Effective Clinical Teacher

Effective Clinical Teacher

- Knowledge of the clinical area.
- Knowledge of clinical teaching.
- Critically diagnose the students' needs.
- Learn about student as individual, their needs, personalities and capabilities.
- Serve as a role model.
- Provide frequent feedback.
- Accept difference among students.

Faculty must serve as resource advisor and source of support

- Clinical learning experience provide opportunity for studies to bridge the gap between theory and practice.
- The assignment for each specialty as per INC and state nursing council requirements, must meet the learning objectives.
- A variety of teaching methods can be used to enable student to acquire desired outcome.

COMMON TERMINOLOGY USED IN NURSING

- **Abduction:** Movement of a body part away from the midline of the body.
- **Activities of daily living (ADL):** The task of daily living such as taking care of personal hygiene, bathing, grooming, eating, exercise, etc.
- **Anger:** An emotional state characterized by the feeling of frustration and struggling with threatening situation.
- **Anxiety:** An emotional state characterized by feeling of uneasiness about the unknown.
- **Asepsis:** Freedom from infection or infectious disease.
- **Auscultation:** Listening to sound produced by different body organ, body structure, created by the movement of air or fluid.
- **Basic human needs:** A basic human need is want of something or requirement for biological, psychological, social or spiritual functioning experienced by a person without which a person cannot survive.
- **Biopsy:** Specimen obtained from a suspicious nodule or the area, using fine needle aspiration or by incision to rule out the diagnosis.
- **Care giver:** The caring or comforting role of the nurse has traditionally included those activities that preserve the dignity of the individual and those often referred to as the mothering actions. In nursing, caring is the role of human relations.
- **Coma:** A state of profound unconsciousness characterized by the absence of spontaneous eye movement, response to painful stimuli and vocalization. The person cannot be awakened.
- **Constant fever:** During a constant fever, the body temperature fluctuates minimally but always remains elevated.
- **Communication:** Communication is the process of exchanging information, thoughts, ideas and feelings from one individual to another.
- **Cyanosis:** Bluish discoloration of the skin and mucous membrane observed in lips, nail beds and ear lobes.
- **Diastolic pressure:** The diastolic pressure is the minimum pressure of the blood against the walls of the vessels following closure of the aortic valve and is taken as direct indication of blood vessels resistance.
- **Digestion:** It is the process by which the food is changed in to simple substances which can be absorbed into the blood.
- **Dose:** The amount of drug given at a time.
- **Catheterization:** Introduction of urethral catheter into the urethra into the urinary bladder to withdraw urine or drain the urine.
- **Edema:** A condition characterized by an excess of water fluid collecting in the body parts.
- **Faith:** Trust in something or someone and belief in a higher power even when there is no evidence or proof.
- **Fear:** An emotional state characterized by expected harm or unpleasantness.
- **Febrile:** Individual suffering with increased body temperature.
- **Fomentation:** A topical treatment of pain or inflammation with a warm moist application.
- **Homeostasis:** A study state within the organ and system in the body.
- **Hypothermia:** Hypothermia is a core of body temperature below the lower limit of normal.
- **Hypoxemia:** Decreased in the arterial oxygen tension in the blood.
- **Incision:** A surgical cut produced by sharp instruments to create an opening into an organ or space in the body.
- **Infection:** It is the entry, development and multiplication of pathogenic microorganisms in the body and cause adverse reaction.
- **Inflammation:** The protective response of the tissues of the body to irritation, injury or infection.
- **Inspection:** Physical examination technique that involves through visual observation.
- **Intermittent fever:** Body temperature alternates at regular intervals between periods of fever and periods of normal temperature.
- **Metabolism:** It refers to all the chemical processes that occurs within a living organism resulting in energy production and growth.
- **Need:** It is a necessity or requirement for life and for wellbeing.

- **Nurse:** A nurse is a person (male or female), who has completed a program on basic nursing education and is qualified and authorized in his/her country to render the most responsible service of a nursing nature, for the promotion and maintenance of the health, and for the prevention of illness and the care of the sick.
- **Nurse-patient relationship:** It is a helping relationship in which the nurse facilitates the health care which is beneficial to him.
- **Nebulization:** Nebulization is the process of administering bronchodilator medication via inhalation delivered into the respiratory tract.
- **Objective data:** Objective data are detectable by the observer or can be tested against on accepted standard, they can be seen, heard, felt, or smelled. *Example:* A discoloration of the skin, blood pressure reading, act of crying known as objective data.
- **Orthopnea:** Orthopnea is shortness of breath that occurs while lying flat and is relieved by sitting or standing.
- **Pain:** It is a feeling of distress, suffering, or agony, caused by stimulation of the sensory nerve ending.
- **Palpation:** Examination of different organs of the body using the sense of touch.
- **Percussion:** The use of sound to examine different organs of the body.
- **Problem:** Problem means an unmet need.
- **Pyrexia:** A body temperature above the usual range is called pyrexia. Fever, a very high temperature, e.g., 41°C (105°F) is called hyperpyrexia.
- **Pulse:** The pulse is a wave of blood created by contraction of the left ventricle of the heart.
- **Range of motion exercise:** Exercises are performed to prevent contractures and joint stiffness by moving all of the joints, muscles through their complete range.
- **Regulating IV flow rate:** During IV infusion monitoring and controlling the rate of intravenous fluid in IV drop factor e.g., 25 drops per minute.
- **Relapsing fever:** In relapsing fever, short febrile period of a few days interferes with periods of 1–2 days of normal temperature.
- **Remittent fever:** Fever in the body temperature fluctuations occurs over the 24 hours period all of which are above normal.
- **Respiration:** Respiration is the act of breathing. It includes the intake of oxygen and the output of carbon dioxide, i.e., respiration consists of inspiration and expiration.
- **Sitz bath:** Sitz bath immersion of the perineal area, hips and buttocks in arm water to relief from discomfort, hemorrhoids, bowel issues and infections.
- **Subjective data:** Subjective data are apparent only to the person affected and can be described or verified only by the person, e.g., itching, pain, known as subjective data.
- **Suture:** A stitch or series of stitches used to close a wound.
- **Systolic pressure:** The systolic pressure is the maximum pressure of the blood against the wall of the vessels following ventricles contraction and is taken as an indication of the integrity of the heart, arteries and arterioles.
- **Tachycardia:** An abnormal condition in which the myocardium contracts regularly but rate is greater than 100 beats per minute.
- **Worry:** A mild form of anxiety characterized by the preoccupation of a problem.
- **Wound:** A wound is a cut or break in the continuity of the skin.
- **Wound swab:** Collection of specimen from a wound.

COMMON INVESTIGATIONS AND THEIR NORMAL VALUES

Sl. No.	Name of the test	Normal value
	Blood count	
1.	Hemoglobin	**Males:** 14.0–17 g/L **Females:** 12.0–16.0 g/L
2.	Erythrocyte sedimentation rate (ESR)	**Male:** 0–15 mm/hr **Female:** 0–20 mm/hr
3.	Leukocyte count (WBC)	**Total:** 4,500–11,000/mm³ **Neutrophils:** 45–73% **Eosinophils:** 0–4% **Basophils:** 0–1% **Lymphocytes:** 20–40% **Monocytes:** 2–8% **Platelet count:** 1,40,000–4,00,000/mm³
4.	Red blood cell (RBC)	14–17 g/dL **Hematocrit (HCT):** Male: 40% Female: 31%
5.	Blood urea	10–50 mg/dL
6.	Serum creatinine	**Female:** 0.6–1.1 mg/dL **Male:** 0.7–1.3 mg/dL
7.	Serum uric acid	2.4–6.0 mg/dL
8.	Serum sodium	3.5–5.1 mEq/L or mmol/L
9.	Serum potassium	**Adult:** 3.5–5.1 mEq/L or mmol/L
10.	Chloride	98–106 mEq/L
11.	Total protein	6.0–8.3 g/dL
12.	Blood normal blood pH	7.35 –7.45
13.	PaO_2	80 –100 mm Hg
14.	$PaCO_2$	35–45 mm Hg
15.	HCO_3	22–26 mm Hg
16.	Saturation O_2	95–99%
17.	Bleeding time	1.5–9.5 minutes
18.	Clotting time	5–8 minutes
19.	Blood urea nitrogen (BUN)	5–15 mg/dL
20.	Prothrombin time	9–12 seconds

Sl. No.	Name of the test	Normal value
21.	Blood chemistries: • Calcium • Creatinine • Magnesium • Potassium • Sodium	8.5 –10.5 mg/dL 0.7–1.4 mg/dL 1.8–3.0 mg/dL 3.5–5 mEq/L 135–145 mEq/L
	Blood sugar	
22.	Blood sugar	**Random blood sugar:** 79–160 mg/dL **FBS:** 70–110 mg/dL **PPBS:** Below 140 mg/dL **GTT:** Fasting 125 mg/dL **1 hour:** <190 mg/dL **2 hour:** 140 mg/dL **3 hour:** 125 mg/dL
23.	Liver function test	**SGOT (AST):** 10–40 IU/L **SGPT (ALT):** 10–40 IU/L **Alkaline phosphate:** 40–112 IU/L **Total protein:** 6–8.5 mg/L **Albumin:** 3.5 –5 g/L **Globulin:** 2–3.5 g/L
24.	Lipid profile	**Total cholesterol:** <200 mg/dL **Triglycerides:** 10–150 mg/dL **HDL cholesterol:** >40–60 mg/dL **LDL cholesterol:** 70–130 mg/dL **VLDL:** ≤2– 30 mg/dL **(0.1–1.7 mmol)** **Lactate dehydrogenase (LDH)** <61 U/mL
25.	HbA1C	**4.5 –6.4:** Excellent control **6.5–7.0:** Good control **7.1 –80:** Acceptable **8.0:** Poor control
26.	Thyroid-stimulating hormone (TSH)	0–15 mIU/L

COMMON EMERGENCY DRUGS

Sl. No.	Name of the drugs	Classification	Adverse reaction	Nursing measure
1.	Aminophylline	Antiasthmatic	Nausea, vomiting, abdominal pain	◆ Maintain adequate hydration ◆ Avoid excessive intake of coffee, tea, and cocoa
2.	Atropine	Muscle relaxants, cardiovascular drugs	Dry mouth, dysphagia, constipation, flushing and dryness of skin	◆ Ensure adequate hydration and frequent mouthwash
3.	Calcium gluconate	Electrolytes	GI Irritation, anorexia, nausea, vomiting, constipation	◆ Advise to take oral calcium 1 hour after meals ◆ Advise to take oral calcium with full glass of water
4.	Diazepam	Anxiolytics	Drowsiness, slurred speech, tremor, headache	◆ Monitor pulse, blood pressure, respiration while administering IV ◆ Tapper dosage gradually
5.	Digoxin	Inotropic	Anorexia, headache, dizziness, drowsiness, convulsions	◆ Monitor apical pulse ◆ Check dosage and preparation carefully
6.	Epinephrine	Sympathomimetic	Drowsiness, headache, nervousness, tremors, dizziness, vertigo	◆ Monitor heart rate ◆ Use extreme caution when calculating and preparing doses
7.	Furosemide	Loop diuretics	Vertigo, headache, dizziness, paresthesia, restlessness, oliguria	◆ Monitor BP after administration ◆ Give early in the day so that increased urination will not disturb sleep
8.	Hydrocortisone	Corticosteroid	Fluid and electrolyte disturbances, muscle weakness, osteoporosis, peptic ulceration	◆ Use minimal doses for minimal duration to minimize adverse effects, tapper doses

NURSING PROCESS

Nursing process is a systematic rational method of planning and providing nursing care. The goal is to identify a client's healthcare status and actual or potential health problems, establish plans to meet the identified needs, and to deliver specific nursing interventions and to address those needs.

■ STEPS IN THE NURSING PROCESS

The nursing process consists of five steps or components. These five steps of the nursing process are assessing, diagnosing, planning, implementing and evaluating. Specific nursing activities and responsibilities are associated with each steps of the nursing process. An overview of the process is as follows:

- **Assessment:** It is collecting, verifying, and organizing data about the client's health status. Data about the physical, emotional, development, social, cultural, intellectual and spiritual aspects of the clients are obtained from a variety of sources.
- **Diagnosis:** It is process of making a clinical judgment (nursing diagnosis) about a client's potential or actual health problem.
- **Planning:** It involves a series of steps in which the nurse and client set priorities, formulate goals or expected outcomes and establish a written care plan for nursing interventions.
- **Implementation:** It is putting the nursing care plan into action.
- **Evaluation:** It is assessing the client's response to predetermined standards. These standards are often referred to as "outcome criteria". If the goals have not been met; reassessment of the care plan is needed.

Nursing assessment	Diagnosis	Goals/ objectives	Planning	Intervention	Scientific principles	Evaluation
♦ It is collecting, verifying and organizing data about a client health status. ♦ Data about the physical, emotional, develo-pmental, social, cultural and spiritual aspects of the client are obtained from a variety of sources.	♦ It is the process of making clinical judgment (nursing diagnosis) about client potential or actual health problem. ♦ In this phase the nurse sorts and clusters the data and analyze what are the actual and potential health problems for which the client needs nursing care.	Goals are declarations of what must be done and are derived from the diagnosis. Established both short– and long–term goals.	♦ What need to be done? ♦ How to be carried out? ♦ Who has to carry out? ♦ Arranging situation to carry out the interv-ention. ♦ Develop specific interv-entions for each nursing diagnosis.	♦ It is putting the nursing care plan into action. ♦ Carrying out the nursing intervention.	Principles underlying Intervention	♦ It is assessing the clients' response to nursing intervention and then comparing the response to predet-ermined standards. ♦ These standards are often referred to as outcome criteria. ♦ If the goal have not been achieved reassessment of the care plan is needed.

■ STUDENT NURSING CARE PLAN

Examples of Nursing Diagnosis and Intervention

Nursing Diagnosis 1

Disturbed sleep pattern:
- **Goal/objectives:** Client will achieve an improved sense of adequate sleep within 2 weeks.
- **Assessment:** Client complaint
  - Having difficulty sleeping
  - It takes hours to falls sleep
  - Client drink 2–3 cuffs coffee after dinner
  - Client has dark circle under eyes
- **Nursing intervention:**
  - Encourage client to establish bedtime routine and regular sleep pattern.
  - Instruct client to limit caffeine, nicotine before bed time.
  - Try to avoid stress (advice relaxation technique).
  - Adjust environment, control noise, temperature, and bright light in bedroom.
  - Avoid daytime sleeping.
  - Advice to read before bedtime.
  - Provide light music.
  - Give warm drink (milk).

Nursing Diagnosis 2

Impaired skin integrity related to pressure and inadequate circulation (patient with pressure ulcer):
- **Goal/objectives:** Client will maintain intact skin, with no further pressure ulcer.
- **Assessment:**
  - Client with pressure ulcer should be assessed for pressure ulcer risk initially on admission and periodic intervals based on the patient condition.
  - Patient should be reassessed every 24 hours and every nurse visit.
  - Observe, moisture, color of the skin changes such as skin that is darker, brownish, bluish, using your hand, ask for then patient for pain sensation.
  - Assess for details of incontinence of urine, feces or both.
- **Nursing intervention:**
  - Use on established risk assessment tool to monitor risk factors.
  - Remove excessive moisture on the skin.
  - Avoid massaging over bony prominence area.
  - Change of position every 2–4 hours to avoid prolonged pressure in one area.
  - Position with pillow to elevate pressure point.
  - Utilize special beds and matters as needed. *Example:* water matters.
  - Instruct client to maintain healthy weight after discharge.
  - Provide ulcer care.

Nursing Diagnosis 3

Altered comfort, pain:
- **Goal:** Client will report (pain reduced) no pain.
- **Assessment:**

  Assess common characteristics of pain:
  - Location: Ask the client to tell the point to all areas of discomfort use anatomical landmark.
  - Intensity: Ask to describe as mild moderate or severe.
  - Pain pattern, relief measure, contributing symptoms.

- **Nursing intervention:**
  - Advised to select nonpharmacological intervention.
  - Administer analgesics if prescribed.
  - Make comfortable sitting position, back resting, keep leg separated, and keep head aligned with spine by using a small thin pillow.
  - Provide cutaneous stimulation to relieve pain, like a massage, warm bath, ice bag, touch and massage.

Nursing Diagnosis 4

Ineffective peripheral tissue perfusion related to improper diabetic foot care and nail hygiene practices (ineffective health maintenance):

- **Goal:**
  - Client peripheral circulation will improve in both feet.
  - Skin integrity in both feet will improve within a month.
- **Nursing intervention:**
  - Discuss with client how to assess feet for breaks in skin friction from shoes and how to avoid foot injury.
  - Instruct client to observe feet for reddened areas, abrasions, blisters and swollen areas immediately after removing shoes.
  - Demonstrate how to clean and apply moisturizers and other skin care product to feet daily.
  - Inform client should see a diabetologist frequently.
  - Refer client to orthotic footwear specialist.
- **Evaluation:**
  - Observe client feet, observe whether blisters are healed, toenail are cleaned and properly trimmed.
  - Client says he observe feet daily after removing shoes and immediately before bed.
  - Client correctly washes and moisturize the feet.

GNM FIRST YEAR

Sl. No.	Practical Record	Requirement
1.	Nursing care plan	4 in medical/surgical wards
2.	Daily diary	1 each in urban and rural community field
3.	a. Health talk b. Family study c. Health assessment of an Individual in the family d. Community profile	1 each urban and rural community field 1 each in urban and rural community field 1 each in urban and rural community field 1 each in urban and rural community field

NURSING CARE PLAN: 1

■ HISTORY TAKING AND PHYSICAL EXAMINATION

Nursing History

Name of the ward: ________________________ Student name: ________________________

Period from: ________________to ____________ Name of the hospital: ________________________

Demographic Data

Name of the patient:	IP No:
Age:	Gender:
Marital status:	Nationality:
Language spoken:	Religion:
Occupation:	Education:
Income:	Address:
Date of admission:	Treatment received on arrival to hospital:
Provisional diagnosis:	Treatment received by patient on arrival:

History of Present Illness

Ask any or all of the following as appropriate and write a summary

Reason for visit: ________________________

When did the symptoms started: ________________________

General state of health: ________________________

Was the onset sudden or gradual: ________________________

How often the problem occurs: ________________________

Has the problem occur before: ________________________

Treatment received on arrival to hospital: ________________________

Chief Complaint

Eliciting a client's history not only assists with individualizing the plan of care but also help to establish a bond with that client.

Gather specific information regarding:

Onset: ________________________.

Location: ________________________.

Duration: ________________________.

Aggravating factors: ________________________.

Relieving factors: ________________________.

Associated manifestation: ____.

Past surgical history: ____.

Past medical history: ____.

Allergies: ____.

Medication History

Medication prescribed. Use of antihypertensive/diuretics/vasodilator/nitroglycerin/anticoagulant/dioxin/bronchodilators/contraceptive/hormones/steroids/antidepressant/psychotropic/thyroid hormones/over the counter medication/herbs note time and dosage and how often they are taking.

____

____

____

Allergies: Note and describe any environmental, food or drug allergies

____

Family History

Type of family: Nuclear/Joint family

Family Composition

Sl. No.	Name	Relationship to the patient	Age	Sex	Education	Occupation	Health status

Family Tree

Family History of Illness

Is there any family history of: Asthma/cancer/diabetes/epilepsy/hypertension/heart disease/hepatitis/hemophilia/stroke/tuberculosis/mental disorders/thyroid or autoimmune disorders/aged grandparent and siblings alive? If yes, what is their current state of health? If no, state the cause of death and age of death _______________________

____

Past Health History

- Previous hospitalization: ____

- Surgery if any: ____

- History of accident or blood transfusion: ____________________________________

- Is the client taking any prescription or over-the-counter medications on a regular basis/notice all the medications, how long: ____

____

Values and Beliefs

- What are the client's attitudes/beliefs about hospitalization?

____

- Does he/she have any inappropriate perception of illness?

____

Dietary Habits

Assess excess or deficit caloric intake and client approximate intake of foods, high in sodium, cholesterol, saturated fat, and caffeine.

____

____

■ PHYSICAL EXAMINATION

Use questioning, observation and examination to gather data. Tick items that apply to the client and comment as needed.

Sensation

Eyes:
- Poor vision/blurred vision/eye infection:
- Blindness R/L/eye pain:
- Itching/prosthesis/glasses/contact lens:

Ears: Ringing in ears/discharge/ear infection/loss of hearing R/L/ear pain/itching/hearing aids.

Tongue: Difficulty of taste.

Nose: Frequent colds/nose bleeds/pain/discharge.

Touch: Reduced or tactile perception.

Skin and mucus membranes: Excessive dryness/bruising/jaundice/itching/rash/broken skin/wound/pale/flushed/ poor turgor/change in pigmentation.

Mouth and throat: Sore throat/coated tongue/dental caries/bad breath (halitosis)/bleeding gums/dentures upper/lower.

Hair: Itchy scalp/hygiene poor/dandruff/hair change/loss/excess.

Nails: Colors changes/biting/splitting/clubbing

Respiration

- Rate: ____
- Cough/dyspnea/wheezing/coughs blood (hemoptysis)/cyanosis/pain on breathing/restlessness—smoke (how many per day): _______________________________________

Circulation

- Pulse rate: ___________________________________/min
- Blood pressure: ______________________________mm Hg
- Fatigue/Chest pain/nausea—vomiting/anemia/varicose veins/peripheral pulses/leg swelling/ulcers.

Nutrition

- Weight: _______________________________________
- Height: _______________________________________
- Skin fold thickness: ___________________________
- Appetite change/weight change/nausea/vomiting/dysphasia/heart burn/dentures/normal eating pattern (likes and dislikes):_______________________________________

Abdomen

- **Inspection:** Rashes/lesions/scar/striae
- **Distended peristalsis:** Present/absent
- **Palpation:** Pain/tenderness/mass

Elimination

Urinary/frequency/urgency/dribbling/urinary incontinence/painful urination retention/dysuria/urinary appliance/ nocturia/hematuria/anuria/distended bladder

Activity/Exercise

Muscle Pain/muscle weakness/cramps/joint pain/swelling/stiffness of movements/deformities/abnormal gait/fatigue/ impaired coordination

Self-care (describe limitation to eating, bathing, dressing, toileting, ambulating) ________________________

____

Comfort

Describes the following:

Pain? If yes, how it is relieved?: ____

Sleep pattern and methods/treatment used for sleep: ________________________________

Neurological Responses

Disorientation/unconscious/headache/tremors/paralysis numbness/weakness/seizures (fits)/dizziness/loss of memory/ difficult expressing self verbally.

Immune Response

- Temperature: ________________________________
- Allergies: ________________________________
- Fever in last 45 hours: ________________________________
- Swollen glands: ________________________________
- COMMENTS: ________________________________

Sexuality

Female:
- Age of menarche: ________________________________
- LMP: ________________________________
- Duration: ________________________________
- Flow: ________________________________
- Cycle: ________________________ days)/dysmenorrheal/bleeding between periods/vaginal bleeding.

Male:

Discharge/swelling/masses; comments: ________________________________

Investigation Done

Date	Name of the investigation	Normal values	Patients values/result	Significance

Medical diagnosis (Final): ________________________________

Drug Management

Name of the drug	Dosage and frequency	Side effect	Nursing intervention

Diet Plan

Type of diet required (snacks, lunch, dinner):

____

____

____

____

____

____

____

____

____

____

____

Nursing Care Plan

ASSESSMENT Subjective Objective	Nursing diagnosis	GOALS Short-term Long-term	Implementation	Evaluation

Summary/Conclusion

Health Education

Reference

Date of submission: **Signature of subject In-charge**

NURSING CARE PLAN: 2

■ HISTORY TAKING AND PHYSICAL EXAMINATION

Nursing History

Name of the ward: ___________________________ Student name: _______________________

Period from: _______________to _______________ Name of the hospital: _______________

Demographic Data

Name of the patient:	IP No:
Age:	Gender:
Marital status:	Nationality:
Language spoken:	Religion:
Occupation:	Education:
Income:	Address:
Date of admission:	Treatment received on arrival to hospital:
Provisional diagnosis:	Treatment received by patient on arrival:

History of Present Illness

Ask any or all of the following as appropriate and write a summary

Reason for visit: ____

When did the symptoms started: ____

General state of health: ____

Was the onset sudden or gradual: ____

How often the problem occurs: ____

Has the problem occur before: ____

Treatment received on arrival to hospital: ____

Chief Complaint

Eliciting a client's history not only assists with individualizing the plan of care but also help to establish a bond with that client.

Gather specific information regarding:

Onset: ____.

Location: ____.

Duration: ____.

Aggravating factors: ____.

Relieving factors: ____.

Associated manifestation: ____.

Past surgical history: ____.

Past medical history: ____.

Allergies: ____.

Medication History

Medication prescribed. Use of antihypertensive/diuretics/vasodilator/nitroglycerin/anticoagulant/dioxin/bronchodilators/contraceptive/hormones/steroids/antidepressant/psychotropic/thyroid hormones/over the counter medication/herbs note time and dosage and how often they are taking.

____

____

____

Allergies: Note and describe any environmental, food or drug allergies

____

Family History

Type of family: Nuclear/Joint family

Family Composition

Sl. No.	Name	Relationship to the patient	Age	Sex	Education	Occupation	Health status

Family Tree

Family History of Illness

Is there any family history of: Asthma/cancer/diabetes/epilepsy/hypertension/heart disease/hepatitis/hemophilia/stroke/tuberculosis/mental disorders/thyroid or autoimmune disorders/aged grandparent and siblings alive? If yes, what is their current state of health? If no, state the cause of death and age of death ___________________________

____

Past Health History

- Previous hospitalization: ____
- Surgery if any: ____
- History of accident or blood transfusion: ____
- Is the client taking any prescription or over-the-counter medications on a regular basis/notice all the medications, how long: ____

____

Values and Beliefs

- What are the client's attitudes/beliefs about hospitalization?

____

- Does he/she have any inappropriate perception of illness?

____

Dietary Habits

Assess excess or deficit caloric intake and client approximate intake of foods, high in sodium, cholesterol, saturated fat, and caffeine.

____

____

■ PHYSICAL EXAMINATION

Use questioning, observation and examination to gather data. Tick items that apply to the client and comment as needed.

Sensation

Eyes:
- Poor vision/blurred vision/eye infection:
- Blindness R/L/eye pain:
- Itching/prosthesis/glasses/contact lens:

Ears: Ringing in ears/discharge/ear infection/loss of hearing R/L/ear pain/itching/hearing aids.

Tongue: Difficulty of taste.

Nose: Frequent colds/nose bleeds/pain/discharge.

Touch: Reduced or tactile perception.

Skin and mucus membranes: Excessive dryness/bruising/jaundice/itching/rash/broken skin/wound/pale/flushed/poor turgor/change in pigmentation.

Mouth and throat: Sore throat/coated tongue/dental caries/bad breath (halitosis)/bleeding gums/dentures upper/lower.

Hair: Itchy scalp/hygiene poor/dandruff/hair change/loss/excess.

Nails: Colors changes/biting/splitting/clubbing

Respiration

- Rate: _______________________________________
- Cough/dyspnea/wheezing/coughs blood (hemoptysis)/cyanosis/pain on breathing/restlessness—smoke (how many per day): _______________________________________

Circulation

- Pulse rate: _______________________________________/min
- Blood pressure: _______________________________________mm Hg
- Fatigue/Chest pain/nausea—vomiting/anemia/varicose veins/peripheral pulses/leg swelling/ulcers.

Nutrition

- Weight: _______________________________________
- Height: _______________________________________
- Skin fold thickness: _______________________________________
- Appetite change/weight change/nausea/vomiting/dysphasia/heart burn/dentures/normal eating pattern (likes and dislikes): _______________________________________

Abdomen

- **Inspection:** Rashes/lesions/scar/striae
- **Distended peristalsis:** Present/absent
- **Palpation:** Pain/tenderness/mass

Elimination

Urinary/frequency/urgency/dribbling/urinary incontinence/painful urination retention/dysuria/urinary appliance/nocturia/hematuria/anuria/distended bladder

Activity/Exercise

Muscle Pain/muscle weakness/cramps/joint pain/swelling/stiffness of movements/deformities/abnormal gait/fatigue/impaired coordination

Self-care (describe limitation to eating, bathing, dressing, toileting, ambulating) _____________________

____

Comfort

Describes the following:

Pain? If yes, how it is relieved?: ____

Sleep pattern and methods/treatment used for sleep: _________________________________

Neurological Responses

Disorientation/unconscious/headache/tremors/paralysis numbness/weakness/seizures (fits)/dizziness/loss of memory/difficult expressing self verbally.

Immune Response

- Temperature: _____________________________________
- Allergies: _____________________________________
- Fever in last 45 hours: _____________________________________
- Swollen glands: _____________________________________
- COMMENTS: _____________________________________

Sexuality

Female:
- Age of menarche: _____________________________________
- LMP: _____________________________________
- Duration: _____________________________________
- Flow: _____________________________________
- Cycle: _____________________________ days)/dysmenorrheal/bleeding between periods/vaginal bleeding.

Male:
Discharge/swelling/masses; comments: _____________________________________

Investigation Done

Date	Name of the investigation	Normal values	Patients values/result	Significance

Medical diagnosis (Final): _____________________________________

Drug Management

Name of the drug	Dosage and frequency	Side effect	Nursing intervention

Diet Plan

Type of diet required (snacks, lunch, dinner):

Nursing Care Plan

ASSESSMENT Subjective Objective	Nursing diagnosis	GOALS Short-term Long-term	Implementation	Evaluation

Summary/Conclusion

Health Education

Reference

Date of submission: **Signature of subject In-charge**

NURSING CARE PLAN: 3

■ HISTORY TAKING AND PHYSICAL EXAMINATION

Nursing History

Name of the ward: _________________________ Student name: _________________________

Period from: _______________ to _______________ Name of the hospital: _________________________

Demographic Data

Name of the patient:	IP No:
Age:	Gender:
Marital status:	Nationality:
Language spoken:	Religion:
Occupation:	Education:
Income:	Address:
Date of admission:	Treatment received on arrival to hospital:
Provisional diagnosis:	Treatment received by patient on arrival:

History of Present Illness

Ask any or all of the following as appropriate and write a summary

Reason for visit: _________________________

When did the symptoms started: _________________________

General state of health: _________________________

Was the onset sudden or gradual: _________________________

How often the problem occurs: _________________________

Has the problem occur before: _________________________

Treatment received on arrival to hospital: _________________________

Chief Complaint

Eliciting a client's history not only assists with individualizing the plan of care but also help to establish a bond with that client.

Gather specific information regarding:

Onset: _________________________.

Location: _________________________.

Duration: _________________________.

Aggravating factors: _________________________.

Relieving factors: _________________________.

Associated manifestation: _________________________.

Past surgical history: _________________________.

Past medical history: _________________________.

Allergies: _________________________.

Medication History

Medication prescribed. Use of antihypertensive/diuretics/vasodilator/nitroglycerin/anticoagulant/dioxin/bronchodilators/contraceptive/hormones/steroids/antidepressant/psychotropic/thyroid hormones/over the counter medication/herbs note time and dosage and how often they are taking.

____

____

Allergies: Note and describe any environmental, food or drug allergies

____

Family History

Type of family: Nuclear/Joint family

Family Composition

Sl. No.	Name	Relationship to the patient	Age	Sex	Education	Occupation	Health status

Family Tree

Family History of Illness

Is there any family history of: Asthma/cancer/diabetes/epilepsy/hypertension/heart disease/hepatitis/hemophilia/ stroke/tuberculosis/mental disorders/thyroid or autoimmune disorders/aged grandparent and siblings alive? If yes, what is their current state of health? If no, state the cause of death and age of death ___________________________

____

Past Health History

- Previous hospitalization: ____

- Surgery if any: ____

- History of accident or blood transfusion: _______________________________________

- Is the client taking any prescription or over-the-counter medications on a regular basis/notice all the medications, how long: ____

____

Values and Beliefs

- What are the client's attitudes/beliefs about hospitalization?

____

- Does he/she have any inappropriate perception of illness?

____

Dietary Habits

Assess excess or deficit caloric intake and client approximate intake of foods, high in sodium, cholesterol, saturated fat, and caffeine.

____

____

■ PHYSICAL EXAMINATION

Use questioning, observation and examination to gather data. Tick items that apply to the client and comment as needed.

Sensation

Eyes:
- Poor vision/blurred vision/eye infection:
- Blindness R/L/eye pain:
- Itching/prosthesis/glasses/contact lens:

Ears: Ringing in ears/discharge/ear infection/loss of hearing R/L/ear pain/itching/hearing aids.

Tongue: Difficulty of taste.

Nose: Frequent colds/nose bleeds/pain/discharge.

Touch: Reduced or tactile perception.

Skin and mucus membranes: Excessive dryness/bruising/jaundice/itching/rash/broken skin/wound/pale/flushed/ poor turgor/change in pigmentation.

Mouth and throat: Sore throat/coated tongue/dental caries/bad breath (halitosis)/bleeding gums/dentures upper/lower.

Hair: Itchy scalp/hygiene poor/dandruff/hair change/loss/excess.

Nails: Colors changes/biting/splitting/clubbing

Respiration

- Rate: _______________________________
- Cough/dyspnea/wheezing/coughs blood (hemoptysis)/cyanosis/pain on breathing/restlessness—smoke (how many per day): _______________________________

Circulation

- Pulse rate: _______________________________/min
- Blood pressure: _______________________________mm Hg
- Fatigue/Chest pain/nausea—vomiting/anemia/varicose veins/peripheral pulses/leg swelling/ulcers.

Nutrition

- Weight: _______________________________
- Height: _______________________________
- Skin fold thickness: _______________________________
- Appetite change/weight change/nausea/vomiting/dysphasia/heart burn/dentures/normal eating pattern (likes and dislikes):_______________________________

Abdomen

- **Inspection:** Rashes/lesions/scar/striae
- **Distended peristalsis:** Present/absent
- **Palpation:** Pain/tenderness/mass

Elimination

Urinary/frequency/urgency/dribbling/urinary incontinence/painful urination retention/dysuria/urinary appliance/nocturia/hematuria/anuria/distended bladder

Activity/Exercise

Muscle Pain/muscle weakness/cramps/joint pain/swelling/stiffness of movements/deformities/abnormal gait/fatigue/impaired coordination

Self-care (describe limitation to eating, bathing, dressing, toileting, ambulating) _______________________________

____

Comfort

Describes the following:

Pain? If yes, how it is relieved?: _______________________________

Sleep pattern and methods/treatment used for sleep: _______________________________

Neurological Responses

Disorientation/unconscious/headache/tremors/paralysis numbness/weakness/seizures (fits)/dizziness/loss of memory/difficult expressing self verbally.

Immune Response

- Temperature: ____
- Allergies: ____
- Fever in last 45 hours: ____
- Swollen glands: ____
- COMMENTS: ____

Sexuality

Female:
- Age of menarche: ____
- LMP: ____
- Duration: ____
- Flow: ____
- Cycle: _______________________________ days)/dysmenorrheal/bleeding between periods/vaginal bleeding.

Male:
Discharge/swelling/masses; comments: ____

Investigation Done

Date	Name of the investigation	Normal values	Patients values/result	Significance

Medical diagnosis (Final): ____

Drug Management

Name of the drug	Dosage and frequency	Side effect	Nursing intervention

Diet Plan

Type of diet required (snacks, lunch, dinner):

____

____

____

____

____

____

Nursing Care Plan

ASSESSMENT Subjective Objective	Nursing diagnosis	GOALS Short-term Long-term	Implementation	Evaluation

Summary/Conclusion

Health Education

Reference

Date of submission:

Signature of subject In-charge

NURSING CARE PLAN: 4

■ HISTORY TAKING AND PHYSICAL EXAMINATION

Nursing History

Name of the ward: _______________________ Student name: _______________________

Period from: _______________to _______________ Name of the hospital: _______________________

Demographic Data

Name of the patient:	IP No:
Age:	Gender:
Marital status:	Nationality:
Language spoken:	Religion:
Occupation:	Education:
Income:	Address:
Date of admission:	Treatment received on arrival to hospital:
Provisional diagnosis:	Treatment received by patient on arrival:

History of Present Illness

Ask any or all of the following as appropriate and write a summary

Reason for visit:_______________________

When did the symptoms started: _______________________

General state of health: _______________________

Was the onset sudden or gradual: _______________________

How often the problem occurs: _______________________

Has the problem occur before: _______________________

Treatment received on arrival to hospital: _______________________

Chief Complaint

Eliciting a client's history not only assists with individualizing the plan of care but also help to establish a bond with that client.

Gather specific information regarding:

Onset:_______________________.

Location: _______________________.

Duration: _______________________.

Aggravating factors: _______________________.

Relieving factors: _______________________.

Associated manifestation: _______________________.

Past surgical history: _______________________.

Past medical history: _______________________.

Allergies: _______________________.

Medication History

Medication prescribed. Use of antihypertensive/diuretics/vasodilator/nitroglycerin/anticoagulant/dioxin/bronchodilators/contraceptive/hormones/steroids/antidepressant/psychotropic/thyroid hormones/over the counter medication/herbs note time and dosage and how often they are taking.

____.

____

Allergies: Note and describe any environmental, food or drug allergies

____

Family History

Type of family: Nuclear/Joint family

Family Composition

Sl. No.	Name	Relationship to the patient	Age	Sex	Education	Occupation	Health status

Family Tree

Family History of Illness

Is there any family history of: Asthma/cancer/diabetes/epilepsy/hypertension/heart disease/hepatitis/hemophilia/stroke/tuberculosis/mental disorders/thyroid or autoimmune disorders/aged grandparent and siblings alive? If yes, what is their current state of health? If no, state the cause of death and age of death _______________________

Past Health History

- Previous hospitalization: _______________________
- Surgery if any: _______________________
- History of accident or blood transfusion: _______________________
- Is the client taking any prescription or over-the-counter medications on a regular basis/notice all the medications, how long: _______________________

Values and Beliefs

- What are the client's attitudes/beliefs about hospitalization?

- Does he/she have any inappropriate perception of illness?

Dietary Habits

Assess excess or deficit caloric intake and client approximate intake of foods, high in sodium, cholesterol, saturated fat, and caffeine.

■ PHYSICAL EXAMINATION

Use questioning, observation and examination to gather data. Tick items that apply to the client and comment as needed.

Sensation

Eyes:
- Poor vision/blurred vision/eye infection:
- Blindness R/L/eye pain:
- Itching/prosthesis/glasses/contact lens:

Ears: Ringing in ears/discharge/ear infection/loss of hearing R/L/ear pain/itching/hearing aids.

Tongue: Difficulty of taste.

Nose: Frequent colds/nose bleeds/pain/discharge.

Touch: Reduced or tactile perception.

Skin and mucus membranes: Excessive dryness/bruising/jaundice/itching/rash/broken skin/wound/pale/flushed/poor turgor/change in pigmentation.

Mouth and throat: Sore throat/coated tongue/dental caries/bad breath (halitosis)/bleeding gums/dentures upper/lower.

Hair: Itchy scalp/hygiene poor/dandruff/hair change/loss/excess.

Nails: Colors changes/biting/splitting/clubbing

Respiration

- Rate: ____
- Cough/dyspnea/wheezing/coughs blood (hemoptysis)/cyanosis/pain on breathing/restlessness—smoke (how many per day): ____

Circulation

- Pulse rate: _______________________________/min
- Blood pressure: _______________________________mm Hg
- Fatigue/Chest pain/nausea—vomiting/anemia/varicose veins/peripheral pulses/leg swelling/ulcers.

Nutrition

- Weight: _______________________________________
- Height: _______________________________________
- Skin fold thickness: _______________________________
- Appetite change/weight change/nausea/vomiting/dysphasia/heart burn/dentures/normal eating pattern (likes and dislikes):____

Abdomen

- **Inspection:** Rashes/lesions/scar/striae
- **Distended peristalsis:** Present/absent
- **Palpation:** Pain/tenderness/mass

Elimination

Urinary/frequency/urgency/dribbling/urinary incontinence/painful urination retention/dysuria/urinary appliance/nocturia/hematuria/anuria/distended bladder

Activity/Exercise

Muscle Pain/muscle weakness/cramps/joint pain/swelling/stiffness of movements/deformities/abnormal gait/fatigue/impaired coordination

Self-care (describe limitation to eating, bathing, dressing, toileting, ambulating) ____

____

Comfort

Describes the following:

Pain? If yes, how it is relieved?: ____

Sleep pattern and methods/treatment used for sleep: ____

Neurological Responses

Disorientation/unconscious/headache/tremors/paralysis numbness/weakness/seizures (fits)/dizziness/loss of memory/difficult expressing self verbally.

Immune Response

- Temperature: _______________________________
- Allergies: _______________________________
- Fever in last 45 hours: _______________________________
- Swollen glands: _______________________________
- COMMENTS: _______________________________

Sexuality

Female:

- Age of menarche: _______________________________
- LMP: _______________________________
- Duration: _______________________________
- Flow: _______________________________
- Cycle: _______________________________ days)/dysmenorrheal/bleeding between periods/vaginal bleeding.

Male:

Discharge/swelling/masses; comments: _______________________________

Investigation Done

Date	Name of the investigation	Normal values	Patients values/result	Significance

Medical diagnosis (Final): _______________________________

Drug Management

Name of the drug	Dosage and frequency	Side effect	Nursing intervention

Diet Plan

Type of diet required (snacks, lunch, dinner):

____

____

____

____

____

____

Nursing Care Plan

ASSESSMENT Subjective Objective	Nursing diagnosis	GOALS Short-term Long-term	Implementation	Evaluation

Summary/Conclusion

Health Education

Reference

Date of submission: **Signature of subject In-charge**

DAILY DIARY IN URBAN COMMUNITY FIELD

Name of the community area: ____

Student name: ____

Year of study: ____

Date of commencement of study: _______________________ Date of completion: _______________________

Name of health center: ____

■ FAMILY IDENTIFICATION

Name of the head of the family: ____

Address: ____

____

____

Occupation: ____

Education: _______________________________ Total income of the family: _______________________

Religion ____

Type of family: Nuclear/joint/extended

Contact no: ____

■ FAMILY COMPOSITION

Sl. No.	Name of the member	Age and sex	Relationship with head of family	Education/occupation	Health status

■ FAMILY HEALTH STATUS

Regular screening for health practice—followed/not followed: _______________________

Dental checkup—practiced/not practiced: _______________________

Any members of the family suffering from chronic fever. If yes write name, age, diagnosis, (if known), treatment receiving

____

____

____

Does any member have a cough for more than two weeks? _______________________

Does anyone have any other illness (dengue, STD, HIV)? If yes, write detail:_______________________

____

Is there any family history of asthma/cancer/diabetes/epilepsy/hypertension/heart disease/hepatitis/hemophilia/stroke/tuberculosis/mental disorders/thyroid or autoimmune disorders/aged grandparent and sibling alive? If so, what is the current status of health? If not, state the cause of death and age of death.

____

____

____

■ VITAL STATISTICS

Birth Rate

Sl. No.	Date of birth	Sex	Parent's name	Remarks

Death Rate

Sl. No.	Date of death	Sex	Cause of death	Name	Remarks

Marriage Details

Sl. No.	Names of couple	Age	Date of marriage	Remarks

UNDER FIVE CHILDREN

Immunization status of under five children: _______________________________________

____

Specify name, age and reason for not being immunized: _________________________________

____

BCG vaccination: ____

DPT vaccination: ____

Poliomyelitis: ____

Measles vaccination: ____

Vitamin A solution: ____

■ ELIGIBLE COUPLE

Is there any eligible couple, if yes list the details:

____

____

Sl. No.	Name of the couple	Age	Using contraceptive Method	Vasectomy	Tubal ligation	Oral contraceptive

Specify if any couple not interested to adopt Family Planning method (state the reason)

____

____

____

Using contraceptive method, if yes specify: Vasectomy/tubal ligation

____

____

Is any women pregnant? If yes, write the following remarks:

1. Gravida ____

2. Registered in hospital: Yes/no

3. Pregnant women receiving iron and folic acid: Yes/no

4. Women receiving tetanus toxoid________________________

In addition students are expected to obtain following information by observation and other methods:

1. Description of the urban community location.

2. Topography.

3. Climate.

4. History.

5. Maintain record of road to health card knowing the degree of malnutrition for under 5 (use nutritional assessment)

____

Date of survey: **Date of submission:**

Signature of subject In–charge:

NOTE

■ HOME VISIT RESPONSIBILITY

Sl. No.	Responsibility	Task
1.	Previsit preparation	• Identify exact location of home • Prepare for safe visit
2.	Orientation period	• Introduce yourself • Review available family data • Identify family problems
3.	Intervention period	• Assess family needs/problem assessment • Suggest what need to be done as per health needs so the family refer appropriately if needed • Give health teaching/counseling as needed • Assess need for other service • Any illness in the family/treatment receiving/advice as required
4.	Termination period	• Summarize visit activities with family member/individual • Explain next visit

DAILY DIARY IN RURAL COMMUNITY FIELD

Name of the community area: ____

Student name: ____

Year of study: ____

Date of commencement of study: _______________ Date of completion: _______________ Name of health center:

____

■ FAMILY IDENTIFICATION

Name of the head of the family: ____

Address: ____

____

Occupation: ____

Education: ______________________________ Total income of the family: _______________

Religion: ____

Type of family: Nuclear/Joint/Extended

Contact no.: ____

■ FAMILY COMPOSITION

Sl. No.	Name of the member	Relationship with head of the family	Age	Sex	Education	Income	Health status

■ HOUSING AND SANITARY CONDITION

- **Type of house:** Kutcha/pucca/semi-pucca/tiles/own/rented
- **Number of rooms:** _______________________________
- **Number of inhabitants:** _______________________________
- **Sleeping arrangements—provision of privacy:** Yes/No
- **Ventilation:** Adequate/inadequate/no ventilation
- **Wash room facility:** Adequate/inadequate
- **Living space:** Adequate/inadequate
- **Lighting:** Electricity/gas lamp/lamplight
- **Drinking water supply:** Public supply/bore well/open tank
- **Kitchen ventilation and light:** Adequate/inadequate
- **Cooking use:** Fire wood/kerosene/cow dung
- **Toilet type:** Sanitary use—public lavatory/open air defecation
- **Cloth washing facilities:** Adequate/use tank water/open well
- **Drainage system:** Open/closed/soakage/drain/kitchen/garden/pit
- **Is the sullage water being disposed hygienically:** Yes/No
- **Measure to control insects (flies and rodents):** Present/no measure?
- **System of waste disposal:** Disposed hygienically, if yes/no–close to the house/separate from the house/separate from resident area (burning/burying/composing)
- **Open space around the house:** Yes/No
- **Water stagnation:** Yes/No
- Are the cattle and poultry housed hygienically? Yes/No. If yes, Separate/within house.
- Is there a well or hand pump? Yes/No. If yes, is it maintained in good order? Yes/No.
- Are there any stray dogs in the vicinity? Yes/No. If yes, write approximate number of dogs_______________
- **Summary:** Any relevant information: _______________________________
  ____

■ FAMILY HEALTH STATUS

Regular screening for health practice–followed/not followed.

Dental check–up: Practiced/not practiced.

Any members of the family suffering from chronic fever, if yes, write name, age, diagnosis (if known) treatment receiving
____

Does any many member have a cough for more than two weeks? _______________________________

Does any member have skin disease (e.g., Itching, patch write, age, diagnosis and treatment)? _______________________________
____

Does one have any other illness (dengue/HIV/STD)? If yes, write detail: _______________________________
____

Is there any family history of asthma/cancer/diabetes/epilepsy/hypertension/heart disease/hepatitis/hemophilia/stroke/tuberculosis/mental disorders/thyroid/any other? Specify _______________________________
____

Food consumption by the family members (calculate for one day or one week) notes based on the total family income able to meet caloric requirements.

Sl. No.	Breakfast	Mid-morning	Lunch	Evening	Dinner	Total intake of: Carbohydrate__________ Protein_____________ Fat________________

Note selection and preparation of food: ____

Any family member suffering from malnutrition? If yes, take complete nutrition assessment._____________________

____

Is there any child under five in family who shows signs of malnutrition?

Sl. No.	Name	Age	Kwashiorkor	Marasmus	Vitamin A deficiency	Anemia	Rickets

◼ VITAL STATISTICS

Birth Rate

Sl. No.	Date of birth	Sex	Parent's name	Remarks

Death Rate

Sl. No.	Date of death	Sex	Cause of death	Name	Remarks

Marriage Details

Sl. No.	Names of couple	Age	Date of marriage	Remarks

Under Five Children

Immunization status of under five children: _______________________________

Specify name, age and reason for not being immunized: _______________________________
____

BCG vaccination: _______________________________

DPT vaccination: _______________________________

Poliomyelitis: _______________________________

Measles vaccination: _______________________________

Vitamin A solution: _______________________________

Eligible Couple

Is there any eligible couple? If yes, list their name:

Sl. No.	Name of the couple	Age	Using contraceptive method	Vasectomy	Tubal legation	Oral contraceptives
1.						
2.						
3.						
4.						
5.						

Specify if any couple not interested to adopt Family Planning method (state the reason): _______________________________
____
____

If any women pregnant? If yes, write the following:
1. Gravida: _______________________________
2. Registered in the hospital: Yes/No
3. Pregnant women receiving iron and folic acid: Yes/No
4. Women receiving tetanus toxoid: Yes/No

Vulnerable Family Members

Sl. No.	Vulnerable family member for	Name of the member	Number	Health assessment	Problem identified
1.	Under five children				
2.	Antenatal mother				
3.	Lactating mother				
4.	School children				
5.	Adolescent				
6.	Elderly				
7.	Challenging physically and mentally				
8.	Others				

Transport and Communication Media

- Own tempo/tractor/uses private transport:
- TV/Phone:
- Newspaper/magazine:
- Language known: ____
- Dietary pattern of family: ____
- Statement of the expenditure of the family: ____

In addition, students are expected to obtain following information by observation or other method
1. Description of the community location
2. Topography History
3. Number of school
4. No. of healthcare agencies
5. Balwadi or ICDS center
6. Place of worship
7. Maintain record of road to health card for knowing degree of malnutrition for under 5, use nutritional assessment.

Date of survey: **Date of submission:**

Signature of subject In-charge:

HEALTH-TALK IN URBAN COMMUNITY FIELD

Date and time: ___________________ Place: _________________________________

Activities	Remarks by clinical supervisor
Preparation of area	
Group participated and number of participants	
Seating arrangement	
Self–introduction	
Introduction of topic	
Subject matter relevant/adequate	
Adequacy and coverage of content	
Method of teaching	
Clear the doubts of participants	
AV aids used	
Interaction from the participants	
Correct use of terms and language	

Summary of health teaching topic: _______________________________________

____

____

____

____

____

____

____

____

____

____

____

____

Date of submission: **Signature of subject In-charge**

HEALTH-TALK IN RURAL COMMUNITY FIELD

Date and time: ________________________ Place: ________________________

Activities	Remarks by clinical supervisor
Preparation of area	
Group participated and number of participants	
Seating arrangement	
Self-introduction	
Introduction of topic	
Subject matter relevant/adequate	
Adequacy and coverage of content	
Method of teaching	
Clear the doubts of participants	
AV aids used	
Interaction from the participants	
Correct use of terms and language	

Summary of health teaching topic: ________________________

____

____

____

____

____

____

____

____

____

____

____

____

Date of submission: **Signature of subject In-charge:**

FAMILY STUDY IN URBAN COMMUNITY FIELD

Name of the community area: _______________________________________

Student name: _______________________________________

Roll no: _______________________________________

Date of commencement of study: _______________ ·Date of completion: _______________

Name of the health center: _______________________________________

Family Identification

- Name of the head of the family: _______________________________________
- Address: _______________________________________
- Type of family/nuclear/joint/extended: _______________________________________
- Occupation: _______________________________________
- Total income of the family: _______________________________________
- Religion: _______________________________________
- Contact no.: _______________________________________

Family Composition

Sl. No.	Name of the member	Relationship with head of the family	Age	Sex	Education	Income	Health status

Housing and Sanitary Condition

- **Type of house:** Kutcha/pucca/semipucca/tiles/own/rented
- **Number of rooms:** _______________ Number of inhabitants: _______________
- **Sleeping arrangements:** Provision of privacy. Yes/No
- **Ventilation:** Adequate/inadequate/no ventilation.
- **Washroom facility:** Adequate/inadequate.
- **Living space:** Adequate/inadequate.
- **Lighting:** Electricity/gas lamp/lamplight.
- **Drinking water supply:** Public supply/bore well/open tank.
- **Kitchen ventilation and light:** Adequate/inadequate.
- **Cooking use:** Fire wood/kerosene/cow dung.
- **Toilet type–sanitary use:** Public lavatory/open air defecation.

- **Cloth washing facilities:** Adequate/use tank water/open well.
- **Drainage system:** Open/closed/soakage/drain/kitchen/garden/pit.
- **Is the sullage water being disposed hygienically:** Yes/No.
- **Measure to control insects, files and rodents:** Present/No measure.
- **System of waste disposal (disposed hygienically):** If Yes/No—Close to the house/separate from the house/separate from resident area (burning/burying/composing)
- **Open space around the house:** Yes/No.
- **Water stagnation:** Yes/No.
- Are the cattle and poultry housed hygienically? Yes/No. If yes, separate/within house.
- Is there a well or hand pump? Yes/No. If yes, is it maintained in good order? Yes/No.
- Are there any stray dogs in the vicinity? Yes/No. If yes, write approximate number of dogs_______________
- **Summary—any relevant information:** ____
____
____

Family Health Status

- **Regular screening for health practice:** Followed/not followed.
- **Dental check–up:** Practiced/not practiced.
- Any members of the family suffering from chronic fever, if yes, write name, age, diagnosis (if known) treatment receiving:____
- Does any many member have a cough for more than two weeks? _______________________________
- Does any member have skin disease (e.g., Itching, patch write, age, diagnosis and treatment)?
____
- Does one have any other illness (dengue/HIV/STD)? If yes, write detail: _______________________
____
- Is there any family history of asthma/cancer/diabetes/epilepsy/hypertension/heart disease/hepatitis/hemophilia/stroke/tuberculosis/mental disorders/thyroid/any other? Specify _______________________

Food consumption by the family members (calculate for one day or one week) notes based on the total family income able to meet caloric requirements

Sl. No.	Breakfast	Mid-morning	Lunch	Evening	Dinner	Total intake of: Carbohydrate____________ Protein_______________ Fat_________________

Note selection and preparation of food: ____

Any family member suffering from malnutrition, if yes, take complete nutrition assessment: _______________
____

Is there any child under five in family who shows signs of malnutrition?

Sl. No.	Name	Age	Kwashiorkor	Marasmus	Vitamin A deficiency	Anemia	Rickets

■ VITAL STATISTICS

Birth Rate

Sl. No.	Date of birth	Sex	Parent's name	Remarks

Death Rate

Sl. No.	Date of death	Sex	Cause of death	Name	Remarks

Marriage Details

Sl. No.	Names of couple	Age	Date of marriage	Remarks

Under Five Children

Immunization status of under five children: ____

- Specify name, age and reason for not being immunized: _______________________________

  ____

- BCG vaccination: ____
- DPT vaccination: ____
- Poliomyelitis: ____
- Measles vaccination: ____
- Vitamin A solution: ____

Eligible Couple

Is there any eligible couple, if yes list their name:

Sl. No.	Name of the couple	Age	Using contraceptive method	Vasectomy	Tubal ligation	Oral contraceptives

Specify if any couple not interested to adopt Family Planning method (state the reason): ___________

____

____

If any women pregnant? If yes, write the following:

1. Gravida: _______________________________
2. Registered in the hospital: Yes/No
3. Pregnant women receiving iron and folic acid: Yes/No
4. Women receiving tetanus toxoid: Yes/No

Vulnerable Family Members

Sl. No.	Vulnerable family member for	Name of the member	Number	Health assessment	Problem identified
1.	Under 5 children				
2.	Antenatal mother				
3.	Lactating mothers				
4.	School children				
5.	Adolescent				
6.	Elderly				
7.	Challenged physically and mentally				
8.	Others				

Transport and Communication Media

- Own tempo/tractor/uses private transport
- TV/Phone
- Newspaper/magazine
- Postal Service: Yes/No
- Language known: _______________________________
- Dietary pattern of family: _______________________________
- Statement of the expenditure of the family: _______________________________

In addition, students are expected to obtain following information by observation or other method

- Description of the community location
- Topography history
- Number of school
- No. of healthcare agencies
- Balwadi or ICDS center
- Place of worship
- Maintain record of road to health card for knowing degree of malnutrition for under 5, use nutritional assessment.

Date of survey: **Date of submission:**

Signature of Community In-charge teacher:

FAMILY STUDY IN RURAL COMMUNITY FIELD

Name of the community area: ____

Student name: ____

Roll no.: ____

Date of commencement of study: _________________ Date of completion: _____________

Name of the health center: ____

Family Identification

- Name of the head of the family: _______________________________________
- Address: ____
- Type of family/nuclear/joint/extended: _________________________________
- Occupation: ____
- Total income of the family: ____
- Religion: ____
- Contact no.: ____

Family Composition

Sl. No.	Name of the member	Relationship with head of the family	Age	Sex	Education	Income	Health status

Housing and Sanitary Condition

- **Type of house:** Kutcha/pucca/semipucca/tiles/own/rented
- **Number of rooms:** ________________ Number of inhabitants: ________________
- **Sleeping arrangements:** Provision of privacy. Yes/No
- **Ventilation:** Adequate/inadequate/no ventilation.
- **Washroom facility:** Adequate/inadequate.
- **Living space:** Adequate/inadequate.
- **Lighting:** Electricity/gas lamp/lamplight.
- **Drinking water supply:** Public supply/bore well/open tank.
- **Kitchen ventilation and light:** Adequate/inadequate.
- **Cooking use:** Fire wood/kerosene/cow dung.
- **Toilet type-sanitary use:** Public lavatory/open air defecation.
- **Cloth washing facilities:** Adequate/use tank water/open well.
- **Drainage system:** Open/closed/soakage/drain/kitchen/garden/pit.
- **Is the sullage water being disposed hygienically:** Yes/No.

- **Measure to control insects, files and rodents:** Present/No measure.
- **System of waste disposal (disposed hygienically):** If Yes/No—Close to the house/separate from the house/separate from resident area (burning/burying/composing)
- **Open space around the house:** Yes/No.
- **Water stagnation:** Yes/No.
- Are the cattle and poultry housed hygienically? Yes/No. If yes, separate/within house.
- Is there a well or hand pump? Yes/No. If yes, is it maintained in good order? Yes/No.
- Are there any stray dogs in the vicinity? Yes/No. If yes, write approximate number of dogs: _______________
- **Summary—any relevant information:** _______________
- _______________

Family Health Status

- Regular screening for health practice: Followed/not followed.
- Dental check–up: Practiced/not practiced.
- Any members of the family suffering from chronic fever, if yes, write name, age, diagnosis (if known) treatment receiving

____

- Does any many member have a cough for more than two weeks? _______________
- Does any member have skin disease (e.g., Itching, patch write, age, diagnosis and treatment)? _______________
- Does one have any other illness (dengue/HIV/STD)? If yes, write detail: _______________
- Is there any family history of asthma/cancer/diabetes/epilepsy/hypertension/heart disease/hepatitis/hemophilia/stroke/tuberculosis/mental disorders/thyroid/any other? Specify : _______________

Food consumption by the family members (calculate for one day or one week). Notes based on the total family income able to meet caloric requirements

Sl. No.	Breakfast	Mid-morning	Lunch	Evening	Dinner	Total intake of: Carbohydrate_______ Protein_______ Fat_______

Note selection and preparation of food: _______________

Any family member suffering from malnutrition, if yes take complete nutrition assessment: _______________

Is there any child under five in family who shows signs of malnutrition?

Sl. No.	Name	Age	Kwashiorkor	Marasmus	Vitamin A deficiency	Anemia	Rickets

■ VITAL STATISTICS

Birth Rate

Sl. No.	Date of birth	Sex	Parent's name	Remarks

Death Rate

Sl. No.	Date of death	Sex	Cause of death	Name	Remarks

Marriage Details

Sl. No.	Names of couple	Age	Date of marriage	Remarks

Under Five Children

Immunization status of under five children: ____

- Specify name, age and reason for not being immunized: ___________________________________

  ____

- BCG vaccination: ____

- DPT vaccination: ____

- Poliomyelitis: ____

- Measles vaccination: ____

- Vitamin A solution: ____

Eligible Couple

Is there any eligible couple, if yes list their name:

Sl. No.	Name of the couple	Age	Using contraceptive method	Vasectomy	Tubal ligation	Oral contraceptives

Specify if any couple not interested to adopt Family Planning method (state the reason): ___________

____

If any women pregnant? If yes, write the following:
1. **Gravida:** ____
2. **Registered in the hospital:** Yes/No
3. **Pregnant women receiving iron and folic acid:** Yes/No
4. **Women receiving tetanus toxoid:** Yes/No

Vulnerable Family Members

Sl. No.	Vulnerable family member for	Name of the member	Number	Health assessment	Problem identified
1.	Under 5 children				
2.	Antenatal mother				
3.	Lactating mothers				
4.	School children				
5.	Adolescent				
6.	Elderly				
7.	Challenged physically and mentally				
8.	Others				

Transport and Communication Media

- Own tempo/tractor/uses private transport
- TV/phone
- Newspaper/magazine
- Postal service: Yes/No
- Language known: _________________________________
- Dietary pattern of family: _________________________________
- Statement of the expenditure of the family: _________________________________

In addition, students are expected to obtain following information by observation or other method

- Description of the community location
- Topography history
- Number of school
- No. of healthcare agencies
- Balwadi or ICDS center
- Place of worship
- Maintain record of road to health card for knowing degree of malnutrition for under 5, use nutritional assessment.

Date of survey: **Date of submission:**

Signature of subject In-charge:

HEALTH ASSESSMENT OF AN INDIVIDUAL IN URBAN FAMILY

■ NURSING HISTORY

Name of the community: _______________________________

Student name: _______________________________

Period from: _________________________ to _________________________

■ HISTORY TAKING AND PHYSICAL EXAMINATION

Demographic Data

Name of the patient:	IP No.:
Age:	Gender:
Marital status:	Nationality:
Language spoken:	◆ Religion: _______________________ ◆ Education: _______________________
Occupation: _______________________ Income: _______________________	Address:

■ CHIEF COMPLAINT

Eliciting a client's history not only assist with individualizing the plan of care but also help to establish a bond with that client.

Gather specific information regarding:

Present symptoms: _______________________________

____

Aggravating factors: _______________________________

____

Relieving factors: _______________________________

____

History of Present Illness

Ask any or all of the following as appropriate and write a summary:

- When did the symptoms started: _______________________________
- General state of health: _______________________________
- Was the onset sudden or gradual: _______________________________
- How often the problem occurs: _______________________________
- Has the problem occur before: _______________________________
- Treatment taken, if any: _______________________________

Medication History

Medication prescribed. Use of antihypertensive/diuretics/vasodilator/nitroglycerin/anticoagulant/dioxin/ bronchodilators/contraceptive/hormones/steroids/antidepressant/psychotropic/thyroid hormones/over the counter medication/herbs. Note time and dosage and how often they are taking.

____

____

____

Allergies: Note and describe any environmental, food or drug allergies

____

Family History

Type of family: Nuclear/Joint family

Family Composition

Sl. No.	Name	Relationship to the patient	Age	Sex	Education	Occupation	Health status

Family Tree

Family History of Illness

Is there any family history of: Asthma/cancer/diabetes/epilepsy/hypertension/heart disease/hepatitis/hemophilia/ stroke/tuberculosis/mental disorders/thyroid or autoimmune disorders/aged grandparent and siblings alive? If yes, what is their current state of health? If no, state the cause of death and age of death _______________________

Past Health History

- Previous hospitalization: _______________________
- Surgery if any: _______________________
- History of accident or blood transfusion: _______________________
- Is the client taking any prescription or over the counter medications on a regular basis/notice all the medications, how long: _______________________

Values and Beliefs

What are the client attitudes/beliefs about hospitalization?

Does he/she have any inappropriate perception of illness?

Dietary Habits

Assess excess or deficit caloric intake and client approximate intake of foods, high in sodium, cholesterol, saturated fat, and caffeine.

■ PHYSICAL EXAMINATION

Use questioning, observation and examination to gather data. Tick items that apply to the client and comment as needed.

Sensation

Eyes:
- Poor vision/blurred vision/eye infection:
- Blindness R/L/eye pain:
- Itching/prosthesis/glasses/contact lens:

Ears: Ringing in ears/discharge/ear infection/loss of hearing R/L/ear pain/itching/hearing aids.

Tongue: Difficulty of taste.

Nose: Frequent colds/nose bleeds/pain/discharge.

Touch: Reduced or tactile perception.

Skin and mucus membranes: Excessive dryness/Bruising/jaundice/itching/rash/broken skin/wound/pale/flushed/ poor turgor/change in pigmentation.

Mouth and throat: Sore throat/coated tongue/dental caries/bad breath (halitosis)/bleeding gums/dentures upper/lower.

Hair: Itchy scalp/hygiene poor/dandruff/hair change/loss/excess.

Nails: Colors changes/biting/splitting/clubbing

Respiration

- Rate: ____
- Cough/dyspnea/wheezing/coughs blood (hemoptysis)/cyanosis/pain on breathing/restlessness—smoke (how many per day: ____

Circulation

- Pulse rate: _________________________________ min
- Blood pressure: _________________________________ mm Hg
- Fatigue/chest pain/nausea—vomiting/anemia/varicose veins/peripheral pulses/leg swelling/ulcers.

Nutrition

- Weight: _________________________________
- Height: _________________________________
- Skin fold thickness: _________________________________
- Appetite change/weight change/nausea/vomiting/dysphasia/heart burn/dentures/normal eating pattern (likes and dislikes): _________________________________

Abdomen

- **Inspection:** Rashes/lesions/scar/striae
- **Distended peristalsis:** Present/absent
- **Palpation:** Pain/tenderness/mass

Elimination

Urinary/frequency/urgency/dribbling/urinary incontinence/painful urination retention/dysuria/urinary appliance/nocturia/hematuria/anuria/distended bladder

Activity/Exercise

Muscle pain/muscle weakness/cramps/joint pain/swelling/stiffness of movements/deformities/abnormal gait/fatigue/impaired coordination

Self–care (describe limitation to eating, bathing, dressing, toileting, ambulating): _________________________________

____

Comfort

Describes the following:

Pain? If yes, how it is relieved?: _________________________________

Sleep pattern and methods/treatment used for sleep: _________________________________

Neurological Responses

Disorientation/unconscious/headache/tremors/paralysis numbness/weakness/seizures (fits)/dizziness/loss of memory/difficult expressing self verbally.

Immune Response

- Temperature: _________________________________
- Allergies: _________________________________
- Fever in last 45 hours: _________________________________
- Swollen glands: _________________________________
- COMMENTS : _________________________________

Sexuality

Female:

- Age of menarche: ________________________________
- LMP: ________________________________
- Duration: ________________________________
- Flow: ________________________________
- Cycle: ________________________________days)/dysmenorrheal/bleeding between periods/vaginal bleeding.

Male:

Discharge/swelling/masses, comments: ________________________________

____

____

Diet Plan

Type of diet required (Snacks, lunch, dinner):

____

____

____

____

____

Date of assessment: **Date of submission:**

Signature of subject In-charge:

HEALTH ASSESSMENT OF AN INDIVIDUAL IN RURAL FAMILY

■ NURSING HISTORY

Name of the community: _______________________________

Student name: _______________________________

Period from: _______________ to _______________

■ HISTORY TAKING AND PHYSICAL EXAMINATION

Demographic Data

Name of the patient:	IP No.:
Age:	Gender
Marital status:	Nationality:
Language spoken:	• Religion: _______________________ • Education _______________________
Occupation: _______________ Income: _______________	Address:

Chief Complaint

Eliciting a client's history not only assist with individualizing the plan of care but also help to establish a bond with that client.

Gather specific information regarding:

Present symptoms: _______________________________

Aggravating factors: _______________________________

Relieving factors: _______________________________

History of Present Illness

Ask any or all of the following as appropriate and write a summary:
- When did the symptoms started: _______________________
- General state of health: _______________________
- Was the onset sudden or gradual: _______________________
- How often the problem occurs: _______________________
- Has the problem occur before: _______________________
- Treatment taken, if any: _______________________

Medication History

Medication prescribed. Use of antihypertensive/diuretics/vasodilator/nitroglycerin/anticoagulant/dioxin/broncho-dilators/contraceptive/hormones/steroids/antidepressant/psychotropic/thyroid hormones/over the counter medication/herbs. Note time and dosage and how often they are taking.

____

____

____

Allergies: Note and describe any environmental, food or drug allergies

____

Family History:

Type of family: Nuclear/Joint family

Family Composition

Sl. No.	Name	Relationship to the patient	Age	Sex	Education	Occupation	Health status

**Family Tree

Family History of Illness

> **Is there any family history of:** Asthma/cancer/diabetes/epilepsy/hypertension/heart disease/hepatitis/hemophilia/stroke/tuberculosis/mental disorders/thyroid or autoimmune disorders/aged grandparent and siblings alive? If yes, what is their current state of health? If no, state the cause of death and age of death ________________________

Past Health History

- Previous hospitalization: ________________________
- Surgery if any: ________________________
- History of accident or blood transfusion: ________________________
- Is the client taking any prescription or over the counter medications on a regular basis/notice all the medications, how long: ________________________

Values and Beliefs

What are the client attitudes/beliefs about hospitalization?

Does he/she have any inappropriate perception of illness?

Dietary Habits

Assess excess or deficit caloric intake and client approximate intake of foods, high in sodium, cholesterol, saturated fat, and caffeine.

■ PHYSICAL EXAMINATION

Use questioning, observation and examination to gather data. Tick items that apply to the client and comment as needed.

Sensation

Eyes:
- Poor vision/blurred vision/eye infection:
- Blindness R/L/eye pain:
- Itching/prosthesis/glasses/contact lens:

Ears: Ringing in ears/discharge/ear infection/loss of hearing R/L/ear pain/Itching/hearing Aids.

Tongue: Difficulty of taste.

Nose: Frequent Colds/nose bleeds/pain/discharge.

Touch: Reduced or tactile perception.

Skin and mucus membranes: Excessive dryness/bruising/jaundice/itching/rash/broken skin/wound/pale/flushed/poor turgor/change in pigmentation.

Mouth and throat: Sore throat/coated tongue/dental caries/bad breath (halitosis)/bleeding gums/dentures upper/lower.

Hair: Itchy scalp/hygiene poor/dandruff/hair change/loss/excess.

Nails: Colors changes/biting/splitting/clubbing

Respiration

- Rate: ____
- Cough/dyspnea/wheezing/coughs blood (hemoptysis)/cyanosis/pain on breathing/restlessness—smoke (how many per day: _______________________________

Circulation

- Pulse rate: _______________________________________min
- Blood pressure: _________________________________mm Hg
- Fatigue/chest pain/nausea—vomiting/anemia/varicose veins/peripheral pulses/leg swelling/ulcers.

Nutrition

- Weight: _______________________________________
- Height: _______________________________________
- Skin fold thickness: _______________________________
- Appetite change/weight change/nausea/vomiting/dysphasia/heart burn/dentures/normal eating pattern (likes and dislikes):____________________________________

Abdomen

- **Inspection:** Rashes/lesions/scar/striae
- **Distended peristalsis:** Present/absent
- **Palpation:** Pain/Tenderness/mass

Elimination

Urinary/frequency/urgency/dribbling/urinary incontinence/painful urination retention/dysuria/urinary appliance/nocturia/hematuria/anuria/distended bladder

Activity/Exercise

Muscle pain/muscle weakness/cramps/joint pain/swelling/stiffness of movements/deformities/abnormal gait/fatigue/impaired coordination

Self-care (describe limitation to eating, bathing, dressing, toileting, ambulating): _______________________

____

Comfort

Describes the following:

Pain? If yes, how it is relieved?: _______________________________

Sleep pattern and methods/treatment used for sleep: _______________________

Neurological Responses

Disorientation/unconscious/headache/tremors/paralysis numbness/weakness/seizures (fits)/dizziness/loss of memory/difficult expressing self verbally.

Immune Response

- Temperature:_______________________________________
- Allergies:____
- Fever in last 45 hours:_______________________________
- Swollen glands:_____________________________________
- COMMENTS:____

Sexuality

Female:

- Age of Menarche:_______________________________
- LMP:_______________________________
- Duration:_______________________________
- Flow:_______________________________
- Cycle: _______________________________(days)/Dysmenorrheal/Bleeding between periods/ Vaginal bleeding.

Male:

Discharge/swelling/masses comments: _______________________________

____

____

Diet Plan

Type of diet required (snacks, lunch, dinner):

____

____

____

____

Date of assessment   **Date of submission**

Signature of subject In-charge

COMMUNITY PROFILE IN URBAN FIELD

Name of the community area: _______________________________________

Student name: _______________________________________

Roll no: _______________________________________

Date of commencement of study: ________________ Date of completion: ________________

Name of the health center: _______________________________________

Family Identification

- Name of the head of the family: _______________________________________
- Address: _______________________________________
- Type of family/nuclear/joint/extended: _______________________________________
- Occupation: _______________________________________
- Total income of the family: _______________________________________
- Religion: _______________________________________
- Contact no.: _______________________________________

Family Composition

Sl. No.	Name of the member	Relationship with head of the family	Age	Sex	Education	Income	Health status

Housing and Sanitary Condition

- **Type of house:** Kutcha/pucca/semipucca/tiles/own/rented
- **Number of rooms:** ________________ Number of inhabitants: ________________
- **Sleeping arrangements:** Provision of privacy. Yes/No
- **Ventilation:** Adequate/inadequate/no ventilation.
- **Washroom facility:** Adequate/inadequate.
- **Living space:** Adequate/inadequate.
- **Lighting:** Electricity/gas lamp/lamplight.
- **Drinking water supply:** Public supply/bore well/open tank.
- **Kitchen ventilation and light:** Adequate/inadequate.
- **Cooking use:** Fire wood/kerosene/cow dung.
- **Toilet type–sanitary use:** Public lavatory/open air defecation.

- **Cloth washing facilities:** Adequate/use tank water/open well.
- **Drainage system:** Open/closed/soakage/drain/kitchen/garden/pit.
- **Is the sullage water being disposed hygienically:** Yes/No.
- **Measure to control insects, files and rodents:** Present/No measure.
- **System of waste disposal (disposed hygienically):** If Yes/No—Close to the house/separate from the house/separate from resident area (burning/burying/composing)
- **Open space around the house:** Yes/No.
- **Water stagnation:** Yes/No.
- Are the cattle and poultry housed hygienically? Yes/No. If yes, separate/within house.
- Is there a well or hand pump? Yes/No. If yes, is it maintained in good order? Yes/No.
- Are there any stray dogs in the vicinity? Yes/No. If yes, write approximate number of dogs_______________
- **Summary—any relevant information:** ____
____
____

Family Health Status

- **Regular screening for health practice:** Followed/not followed.
- **Dental check–up:** Practiced/not practiced.
- Any members of the family suffering from chronic fever, if yes, write name, age, diagnosis (if known) treatment receiving:____
- Does any many member have a cough for more than two weeks? _______________________________
- Does any member have skin disease (e.g., Itching, patch write, age, diagnosis and treatment)?
____
- Does one have any other illness (dengue/HIV/STD)? If yes, write detail: ___________________________
____
- Is there any family history of asthma/cancer/diabetes/epilepsy/hypertension/heart disease/hepatitis/hemophilia/ stroke/tuberculosis/mental disorders/thyroid/any other? Specify ________________________________

Food consumption by the family members (calculate for one day or one week) notes based on the total family income able to meet caloric requirements

Sl. No.	Breakfast	Mid-morning	Lunch	Evening	Dinner	Total intake of: Carbohydrate___________ Protein_______________ Fat________________

Note selection and preparation of food: ____

Any family member suffering from malnutrition, if yes, take complete nutrition assessment:_______________
____

Is there any child under five in family who shows signs of malnutrition?

Sl. No.	Name	Age	Kwashiorkor	Marasmus	Vitamin A deficiency	Anemia	Rickets

■ VITAL STATISTICS

Birth Rate

Sl. No.	Date of birth	Sex	Parent's name	Remarks

Death Rate

Sl. No.	Date of death	Sex	Cause of death	Name	Remarks

Marriage Details

Sl. No.	Names of couple	Age	Date of marriage	Remarks

Under Five Children

Immunization status of under five children: ________________________

- Specify name, age and reason for not being immunized: ________________

  ____

- BCG vaccination: ____
- DPT vaccination: ____
- Poliomyelitis: ____
- Measles vaccination: ____
- Vitamin A solution: ____

Eligible Couple

Is there any eligible couple, if yes list their name:

Sl. No.	Name of the couple	Age	Using contraceptive method	Vasectomy	Tubal ligation	Oral contraceptives

Specify if any couple not interested to adopt Family Planning method (state the reason): ________________

____

If any women pregnant? If yes, write the following:
1. Gravida: _______________________________________
2. Registered in the hospital: Yes/No
3. Pregnant women receiving iron and folic acid: Yes/No
4. Women receiving tetanus toxoid: Yes/No

Vulnerable Family Members

Sl. No.	Vulnerable family member for	Name of the member	Number	Health assessment	Problem identified
1.	Under 5 children				
2.	Antenatal mother				
3.	Lactating mothers				
4.	School children				
5.	Adolescent				
6.	Elderly				
7.	Challenged physically and mentally				
8.	Others				

Transport and Communication Media

- Own tempo/tractor/uses private transport
- TV/Phone
- Newspaper/magazine
- Postal Service: Yes/No
- Language known: _______________________________________
- Dietary pattern of family: _______________________________________
- Statement of the expenditure of the family: _______________________________________

In addition, students are expected to obtain following information by observation or other method

- Description of the community location
- Topography history
- Number of school
- No. of healthcare agencies
- Balwadi or ICDS center
- Place of worship
- Maintain record of road to health card for knowing degree of malnutrition for under 5, use nutritional assessment.

Date of survey: **Date of submission:**

Signature of Community In-charge teacher:

COMMUNITY PROFILE IN RURAL FIELD

Name of the community area: _______________________________

Student name: _______________________________

Roll no.: _______________________________

Date of commencement of study: _______________ Date of completion: _______________

Name of the health center: _______________________________

Family Identification

- Name of the head of the family:_______________________________
- Address: _______________________________
- Type of family/nuclear/joint/extended:_______________________________
- Occupation: _______________________________
- Total income of the family: _______________________________
- Religion: _______________________________
- Contact no.: _______________________________

Family Composition

Sl. No.	Name of the member	Relationship with head of the family	Age	Sex	Education	Income	Health status

Housing and Sanitary Condition

- **Type of house:** Kutcha/pucca/semipucca/tiles/own/rented
- **Number of rooms:** _______________ Number of inhabitants: _______________
- **Sleeping arrangements:** Provision of privacy. Yes/No
- **Ventilation:** Adequate/inadequate/no ventilation.
- **Washroom facility:** Adequate/inadequate.
- **Living space:** Adequate/inadequate.
- **Lighting:** Electricity/gas lamp/lamplight.
- **Drinking water supply:** Public supply/bore well/open tank.
- **Kitchen ventilation and light:** Adequate/inadequate.
- **Cooking use:** Fire wood/kerosene/cow dung.
- **Toilet type–sanitary use:** Public lavatory/open air defecation.
- **Cloth washing facilities:** Adequate/use tank water/open well.
- **Drainage system:** Open/closed/soakage/drain/kitchen/garden/pit.
- **Is the sullage water being disposed hygienically:** Yes/No.

- **Measure to control insects, files and rodents:** Present/No measure.
- **System of waste disposal (disposed hygienically):** If Yes/No—Close to the house/separate from the house/separate from resident area (burning/burying/composing)
- **Open space around the house:** Yes/No.
- **Water stagnation:** Yes/No.
- Are the cattle and poultry housed hygienically? Yes/No. If yes, separate/within house.
- Is there a well or hand pump? Yes/No. If yes, is it maintained in good order? Yes/No.
- Are there any stray dogs in the vicinity? Yes/No. If yes, write approximate number of dogs: ________________
- **Summary—any relevant information:** ________________________________

____

____

Family Health Status

- Regular screening for health practice: Followed/not followed.
- Dental check–up: Practiced/not practiced.
- Any members of the family suffering from chronic fever, if yes, write name, age, diagnosis (if known) treatment receiving

  ____

- Does any many member have a cough for more than two weeks? ________________
- Does any member have skin disease (e.g., Itching, patch write, age, diagnosis and treatment)? ________________
- Does one have any other illness (dengue/HIV/STD)? If yes, write detail:________________
- Is there any family history of asthma/cancer/diabetes/epilepsy/hypertension/heart disease/hepatitis/hemophilia/ stroke/tuberculosis/mental disorders/thyroid/any other? Specify :________________

  ____

Food consumption by the family members (calculate for one day or one week). Notes based on the total family income able to meet caloric requirements

Sl. No.	Breakfast	Mid-morning	Lunch	Evening	Dinner	Total intake of: Carbohydrate________ Protein____________ Fat______________

Note selection and preparation of food: ____

Any family member suffering from malnutrition, if yes take complete nutrition assessment:________________

____

Is there any child under five in family who shows signs of malnutrition?

Sl. No.	Name	Age	Kwashiorkor	Marasmus	Vitamin A deficiency	Anemia	Rickets

■ VITAL STATISTICS

Birth Rate

Sl. No.	Date of birth	Sex	Parent's name	Remarks

Death Rate

Sl. No.	Date of death	Sex	Cause of death	Name	Remarks

Marriage Details

Sl. No.	Names of couple	Age	Date of marriage	Remarks

Under Five Children

Immunization status of under five children: ____

- Specify name, age and reason for not being immunized: ________________________________

  ____

- BCG vaccination: ____
- DPT vaccination: ____
- Poliomyelitis: ____
- Measles vaccination: ____
- Vitamin A solution: ____

Eligible Couple

Is there any eligible couple, if yes list their name:

Sl. No.	Name of the couple	Age	Using contraceptive method	Vasectomy	Tubal ligation	Oral contraceptives

Specify if any couple not interested to adopt Family Planning method (state the reason): ____________

____

If any women pregnant? If yes, write the following:

1. **Gravida:** ____
2. **Registered in the hospital:** Yes/No
3. **Pregnant women receiving iron and folic acid:** Yes/No
4. **Women receiving tetanus toxoid:** Yes/No

Vulnerable Family Members

Sl. No.	Vulnerable family member for	Name of the member	Number	Health assessment	Problem identified
1.	Under 5 children				
2.	Antenatal mother				
3.	Lactating mothers				
4.	School children				
5.	Adolescent				
6.	Elderly				
7.	Challenged physically and mentally				
8.	Others				

Transport and Communication Media

- Own tempo/tractor/uses private transport
- TV/phone
- Newspaper/magazine
- Postal service: Yes/No
- Language known: ___________________________________
- Dietary pattern of family: _______________________________
- Statement of the expenditure of the family: ____

In addition, students are expected to obtain following information by observation or other method

- Description of the community location
- Topography history
- Number of school
- No. of healthcare agencies
- Balwadi or ICDS center
- Place of worship
- Maintain record of road to health card for knowing degree of malnutrition for under 5, use nutritional assessment.

Date of survey: **Date of submission:**

Signature of subject In-charge:

GNM SECOND YEAR

■ SECOND YEAR

Sl. No.	Practical Record	Requirement
1.	**Medical ward**	
	Nursing care plan	2
	Case study	1
	Case presentation	1
	Drug study	1
2.	**Surgical ward**	
	Nursing care plan	2
	Case study	1
	Case presentation	1
	Drug study	1
3.	**Psychiatry ward**	
	Nursing care plan	1
	Case study	1
	Case presentation	1
	Drug study	1
	Process recording	2
	Mental status examination	4
4.	**Pediatric ward**	
	Nursing care plan	2
	Case study	1
	Case presentation	1
	Drug study	1
	Observation report (newborn)	2

MEDICAL WARD

NURSING CARE PLAN: 1

■ HISTORY TAKING AND PHYSICAL EXAMINATION

Nursing History

Name of the ward: _________________________ Student name: _______________________

Period from: ________________to _____________ Name of the hospital: ___________________

Demographic Data

Name of the patient:	IP No:
Age:	Gender:
Marital status:	Nationality:
Language spoken:	Religion:
Occupation:	Education:
Income:	Address:
Date of admission:	Treatment received on arrival to hospital:
Provisional diagnosis:	Treatment received by patient on arrival:

History of Present Illness

Ask any or all of the following as appropriate and write a summary

Reason for visit: ____

When did the symptoms started: ___________________________________

General state of health: ____

Was the onset sudden or gradual: _________________________________

How often the problem occurs: ____________________________________

Has the problem occur before: ____________________________________

Treatment received on arrival to hospital: _________________________

Chief Complaint

Eliciting a client's history not only assists with individualizing the plan of care but also help to establish a bond with that client.

Gather specific information regarding:

Onset: ____.

Location: ____.

Duration: ____.

Aggravating factors: ____.

Relieving factors: ____.

Associated manifestation: ____.

Past surgical history: ____.

Past medical history: ____.

Allergies: ____.

Medication History

Medication prescribed. Use of antihypertensive/diuretics/vasodilator/nitroglycerin/anticoagulant/dioxin/bronchodilators/contraceptive/hormones/steroids/antidepressant/psychotropic/thyroid hormones/over the counter medication/herbs note time and dosage and how often they are taking.

____

____

____

Allergies: Note and describe any environmental, food or drug allergies

____

Family History

Type of family: Nuclear/Joint family

Family Composition

Sl. No.	Name	Relationship to the patient	Age	Sex	Education	Occupation	Health status

Family Tree

Family History of Illness
Is there any family history of: Asthma/cancer/diabetes/epilepsy/hypertension/heart disease/hepatitis/hemophilia/stroke/tuberculosis/mental disorders/thyroid or autoimmune disorders/aged grandparent and siblings alive? If yes, what is their current state of health? If no, state the cause of death and age of death _________________________

____

Past Health History

- Previous hospitalization: ____

- Surgery if any: ____

- History of accident or blood transfusion: _______________________________________

- Is the client taking any prescription or over-the-counter medications on a regular basis/notice all the medications, how long: ____

Values and Beliefs

- What are the client's attitudes/beliefs about hospitalization?

____

- Does he/she have any inappropriate perception of illness?

____

Dietary Habits

Assess excess or deficit caloric intake and client approximate intake of foods, high in sodium, cholesterol, saturated fat, and caffeine.

____

____

■ PHYSICAL EXAMINATION

Use questioning, observation and examination to gather data. Tick items that apply to the client and comment as needed.

Sensation

Eyes:
- Poor vision/blurred vision/eye infection:
- Blindness R/L/eye pain:
- Itching/prosthesis/glasses/contact lens:

Ears: Ringing in ears/discharge/ear infection/loss of hearing R/L/ear pain/itching/hearing aids.

Tongue: Difficulty of taste.

Nose: Frequent colds/nose bleeds/pain/discharge.

Touch: Reduced or tactile perception.

Skin and mucus membranes: Excessive dryness/bruising/jaundice/itching/rash/broken skin/wound/pale/flushed/poor turgor/change in pigmentation.

Mouth and throat: Sore throat/coated tongue/dental caries/bad breath (halitosis)/bleeding gums/dentures upper/lower.

Hair: Itchy scalp/hygiene poor/dandruff/hair change/loss/excess.

Nails: Colors changes/biting/splitting/clubbing

Respiration

- Rate: ________________________________
- Cough/dyspnea/wheezing/coughs blood (hemoptysis)/cyanosis/pain on breathing/restlessness—smoke (how many per day): ________________________________

Circulation

- Pulse rate: ________________________/min
- Blood pressure: ________________________mm Hg
- Fatigue/Chest pain/nausea—vomiting/anemia/varicose veins/peripheral pulses/leg swelling/ulcers.

Nutrition

- Weight: ________________________________
- Height: ________________________________
- Skin fold thickness: ________________________________
- Appetite change/weight change/nausea/vomiting/dysphasia/heart burn/dentures/normal eating pattern (likes and dislikes):________________________________

Abdomen

- **Inspection:** Rashes/lesions/scar/striae
- **Distended peristalsis:** Present/absent
- **Palpation:** Pain/tenderness/mass

Elimination

Urinary/frequency/urgency/dribbling/urinary incontinence/painful urination retention/dysuria/urinary appliance/nocturia/hematuria/anuria/distended bladder

Activity/Exercise

Muscle Pain/muscle weakness/cramps/joint pain/swelling/stiffness of movements/deformities/abnormal gait/fatigue/impaired coordination

Self-care (describe limitation to eating, bathing, dressing, toileting, ambulating) _______________________

____

Comfort

Describes the following:

Pain? If yes, how it is relieved?: ____

Sleep pattern and methods/treatment used for sleep: _______________________________________

Neurological Responses

Disorientation/unconscious/headache/tremors/paralysis numbness/weakness/seizures (fits)/dizziness/loss of memory/difficult expressing self verbally.

Immune Response

- Temperature: ______________________________________
- Allergies: ______________________________________
- Fever in last 45 hours: ______________________________________
- Swollen glands: ______________________________________
- COMMENTS: ______________________________________

Sexuality

Female:
- Age of menarche: ______________________________________
- LMP: ______________________________________
- Duration: ______________________________________
- Flow: ______________________________________
- Cycle: ______________________________ days)/dysmenorrheal/bleeding between periods/vaginal bleeding.

Male:

Discharge/swelling/masses; comments: ____

Investigation Done

Date	Name of the investigation	Normal values	Patients values/result	Significance

Medical diagnosis (Final): ____

Drug Management

Name of the drug	Dosage and frequency	Side effect	Nursing intervention

Diet Plan

Type of diet required (snacks, lunch, dinner):

____

____

____

____

____

____

____

____

____

____

Nursing Care Plan

ASSESSMENT Subjective Objective	Nursing diagnosis	GOALS Short-term Long-term	Implementation	Evaluation

Summary/Conclusion

Health Education

Reference

Date of submission: **Signature of subject In-charge**

NURSING CARE PLAN: 2

■ HISTORY TAKING AND PHYSICAL EXAMINATION

Nursing History

Name of the ward: _______________________ Student name: _______________________

Period from: _______________to _______________ Name of the hospital: _______________________

Demographic Data

Name of the patient:	IP No:
Age:	Gender:
Marital status:	Nationality:
Language spoken:	Religion:
Occupation:	Education:
Income:	Address:
Date of admission:	Treatment received on arrival to hospital:
Provisional diagnosis:	Treatment received by patient on arrival:

History of Present Illness

Ask any or all of the following as appropriate and write a summary

Reason for visit: ____

When did the symptoms started: ____

General state of health: ____

Was the onset sudden or gradual: ____

How often the problem occurs: ____

Has the problem occur before: ____

Treatment received on arrival to hospital: ____

Chief Complaint

Eliciting a client's history not only assists with individualizing the plan of care but also help to establish a bond with that client.

Gather specific information regarding:

Onset: ____.

Location: ____.

Duration: ____.

Aggravating factors: ____.

Relieving factors: ____.

Associated manifestation: ____.

Past surgical history: ____.

Past medical history: ____.

Allergies: ____.

Medication History

Medication prescribed. Use of antihypertensive/diuretics/vasodilator/nitroglycerin/anticoagulant/dioxin/bronchodilators/contraceptive/hormones/steroids/antidepressant/psychotropic/thyroid hormones/over the counter medication/herbs note time and dosage and how often they are taking.

____.

____

____

Allergies: Note and describe any environmental, food or drug allergies

____

Family History

Type of family: Nuclear/Joint family

Family Composition

Sl. No.	Name	Relationship to the patient	Age	Sex	Education	Occupation	Health status

Family Tree

Family History of Illness

Is there any family history of: Asthma/cancer/diabetes/epilepsy/hypertension/heart disease/hepatitis/hemophilia/
stroke/tuberculosis/mental disorders/thyroid or autoimmune disorders/aged grandparent and siblings alive? If yes,
what is their current state of health? If no, state the cause of death and age of death ___________________________

____

Past Health History

- Previous hospitalization: ____

- Surgery if any: ____

- History of accident or blood transfusion: ____

- Is the client taking any prescription or over-the-counter medications on a regular basis/notice all the
  medications, how long:____

____

Values and Beliefs

- What are the client's attitudes/beliefs about hospitalization?

____

- Does he/she have any inappropriate perception of illness?

____

Dietary Habits

Assess excess or deficit caloric intake and client approximate intake of foods, high in sodium, cholesterol, saturated fat,
and caffeine.

____

____

■ PHYSICAL EXAMINATION

Use questioning, observation and examination to gather data. Tick items that apply to the client and comment as needed.

Sensation

Eyes:
- Poor vision/blurred vision/eye infection:
- Blindness R/L/eye pain:
- Itching/prosthesis/glasses/contact lens:

Ears: Ringing in ears/discharge/ear infection/loss of hearing R/L/ear pain/itching/hearing aids.

Tongue: Difficulty of taste.

Nose: Frequent colds/nose bleeds/pain/discharge.

Touch: Reduced or tactile perception.

Skin and mucus membranes: Excessive dryness/bruising/jaundice/itching/rash/broken skin/wound/pale/flushed/ poor turgor/change in pigmentation.

Mouth and throat: Sore throat/coated tongue/dental caries/bad breath (halitosis)/bleeding gums/dentures upper/lower.

Hair: Itchy scalp/hygiene poor/dandruff/hair change/loss/excess.

Nails: Colors changes/biting/splitting/clubbing

Respiration

- Rate: _______________________________________
- Cough/dyspnea/wheezing/coughs blood (hemoptysis)/cyanosis/pain on breathing/restlessness—smoke (how many per day): _______________________________________

Circulation

- Pulse rate: _______________________________/min
- Blood pressure: _______________________________mm Hg
- Fatigue/Chest pain/nausea—vomiting/anemia/varicose veins/peripheral pulses/leg swelling/ulcers.

Nutrition

- Weight: _______________________________________
- Height: _______________________________________
- Skin fold thickness: _______________________________
- Appetite change/weight change/nausea/vomiting/dysphasia/heart burn/dentures/normal eating pattern (likes and dislikes): _______________________________________

Abdomen

- **Inspection:** Rashes/lesions/scar/striae
- **Distended peristalsis:** Present/absent
- **Palpation:** Pain/tenderness/mass

Elimination

Urinary/frequency/urgency/dribbling/urinary incontinence/painful urination retention/dysuria/urinary appliance/ nocturia/hematuria/anuria/distended bladder

Activity/Exercise

Muscle Pain/muscle weakness/cramps/joint pain/swelling/stiffness of movements/deformities/abnormal gait/fatigue/impaired coordination

Self-care (describe limitation to eating, bathing, dressing, toileting, ambulating) ________________________

____

Comfort

Describes the following:

Pain? If yes, how it is relieved?: ________________________________

Sleep pattern and methods/treatment used for sleep: ________________________

Neurological Responses

Disorientation/unconscious/headache/tremors/paralysis numbness/weakness/seizures (fits)/dizziness/loss of memory/difficult expressing self verbally.

Immune Response

- Temperature: ________________________________
- Allergies: ________________________________
- Fever in last 45 hours: ________________________________
- Swollen glands: ________________________________
- COMMENTS: ________________________________

Sexuality

Female:
- Age of menarche: ________________________________
- LMP: ________________________________
- Duration: ________________________________
- Flow: ________________________________
- Cycle: ________________________ days)/dysmenorrheal/bleeding between periods/vaginal bleeding.

Male:

Discharge/swelling/masses; comments: ________________________________

Investigation Done

Date	Name of the investigation	Normal values	Patients values/result	Significance

Medical diagnosis (Final): ________________________________

Drug Management

Name of the drug	Dosage and frequency	Side effect	Nursing intervention

Diet Plan

Type of diet required (snacks, lunch, dinner):

____

____

____

____

____

____

____

____

____

____

____

Nursing Care Plan

ASSESSMENT Subjective Objective	Nursing diagnosis	GOALS Short-term Long-term	Implementation	Evaluation

Summary/Conclusion

Health Education

Reference

Date of submission: **Signature of subject In-charge**

CASE STUDY

■ HISTORY TAKING AND PHYSICAL EXAMINATION AND NURSING

Nursing History

Name of the ward: _______________________ Student name: _______________________

Period from: _______________to _______________ Name of the hospital: _______________________

Demographic Data

Name of the patient:	IP No:
Age:	Gender:
Marital status:	Nationality:
Language spoken:	Religion:
Occupation:	Education:
Income:	Address:
Date of admission:	Treatment received on arrival to hospital:
Provisional diagnosis:	Treatment received by patient on arrival:

History of Present Illness

Ask any or all of the following as appropriate and write a summary

Reason for visit: _______________________

When did the symptoms started: _______________________

General state of health: _______________________

Was the onset sudden or gradual: _______________________

How often the problem occurs: _______________________

Has the problem occur before: _______________________

Treatment received on arrival to hospital: _______________________

Chief Complaint

Eliciting a client's history not only assists with individualizing the plan of care but also help to establish a bond with that client.

Gather specific information regarding:

Onset:_______________________.

Location:_______________________.

Duration:_______________________.

Aggravating factors:_______________________.

Relieving factors:_______________________.

Associated manifestation: ____.

Past surgical history: ____.

Past medical history: ____.

Allergies: ____.

Medication History

Medication prescribed. Use of antihypertensive/diuretics/vasodilator/nitroglycerin/anticoagulant/dioxin/bronchodilators/contraceptive/hormones/steroids/antidepressant/psychotropic/thyroid hormones/over the counter medication/herbs note time and dosage and how often they are taking.

____

____

____

Allergies: Note and describe any environmental, food or drug allergies

____

Family History

Type of family: Nuclear/Joint family

Family Composition

Sl. No.	Name	Relationship to the patient	Age	Sex	Education	Occupation	Health status

Family Tree

Family History of Illness
Is there any family history of: Asthma/cancer/diabetes/epilepsy/hypertension/heart disease/hepatitis/hemophilia/stroke/tuberculosis/mental disorders/thyroid or autoimmune disorders/aged grandparent and siblings alive? If yes, what is their current state of health? If no, state the cause of death and age of death _______________________
____

Past Health History

- Previous hospitalization: ____

- Surgery if any: ____

- History of accident or blood transfusion: _______________________________________

- Is the client taking any prescription or over-the-counter medications on a regular basis/notice all the medications, how long:____
____

Values and Beliefs

- What are the client's attitudes/beliefs about hospitalization?
____

- Does he/she have any inappropriate perception of illness?
____

Dietary Habits

Assess excess or deficit caloric intake and client approximate intake of foods, high in sodium, cholesterol, saturated fat, and caffeine.

____

____

■ PHYSICAL EXAMINATION

Use questioning, observation and examination to gather data. Tick items that apply to the client and comment as needed.

Sensation

Eyes:
- Poor vision/blurred vision/eye infection:
- Blindness R/L/eye pain:
- Itching/prosthesis/glasses/contact lens:

Ears: Ringing in ears/discharge/ear infection/loss of hearing R/L/ear pain/itching/hearing aids.

Tongue: Difficulty of taste.

Nose: Frequent colds/nose bleeds/pain/discharge.

Touch: Reduced or tactile perception.

Skin and mucus membranes: Excessive dryness/bruising/jaundice/itching/rash/broken skin/wound/pale/flushed/poor turgor/change in pigmentation.

Mouth and throat: Sore throat/coated tongue/dental caries/bad breath (halitosis)/bleeding gums/dentures upper/lower.

Hair: Itchy scalp/hygiene poor/dandruff/hair change/loss/excess.

Nails: Colors changes/biting/splitting/clubbing

Respiration

- Rate: ____
- Cough/dyspnea/wheezing/coughs blood (hemoptysis)/cyanosis/pain on breathing/restlessness—smoke (how many per day): ____

Circulation

- Pulse rate: _______________________________/min
- Blood pressure: _______________________________mm Hg
- Fatigue/Chest pain/nausea—vomiting/anemia/varicose veins/peripheral pulses/leg swelling/ulcers.

Nutrition

- Weight: ____
- Height: ____
- Skin fold thickness: ____
- Appetite change/weight change/nausea/vomiting/dysphasia/heart burn/dentures/normal eating pattern (likes and dislikes): ____

Abdomen

- **Inspection:** Rashes/lesions/scar/striae
- **Distended peristalsis:** Present/absent
- **Palpation:** Pain/tenderness/mass

Elimination

Urinary/frequency/urgency/dribbling/urinary incontinence/painful urination retention/dysuria/urinary appliance/nocturia/hematuria/anuria/distended bladder

Activity/Exercise

Muscle Pain/muscle weakness/cramps/joint pain/swelling/stiffness of movements/deformities/abnormal gait/fatigue/impaired coordination

Self-care (describe limitation to eating, bathing, dressing, toileting, ambulating) _________________________

____

Comfort

Describes the following:

Pain? If yes, how it is relieved?: ____

Sleep pattern and methods/treatment used for sleep: ____

Neurological Responses

Disorientation/unconscious/headache/tremors/paralysis numbness/weakness/seizures (fits)/dizziness/loss of memory/difficult expressing self verbally.

Immune Response

- Temperature: _________________________________
- Allergies: _________________________________
- Fever in last 45 hours: _________________________________
- Swollen glands: _________________________________
- COMMENTS:_________________________________

Sexuality

Female:
- Age of menarche: _________________________________
- LMP: _________________________________
- Duration: _________________________________
- Flow: _________________________________
- Cycle: _________________________________ days)/dysmenorrheal/bleeding between periods/vaginal bleeding.

Male:

Discharge/swelling/masses; comments: ____

Comparing Theory Knowledge with Present Patient Condition

Knowledge of disease	As per theory knowledge	Present in patient
Definition		
Review related anatomy and physiology		

Knowledge of disease	As per theory knowledge	Present in patient
Etiology		
Diagnosis		
Clinical manifestation		
Diagnosis evaluation/investigation		
Medical management		
Surgical management		
Dietary management		

Nursing Care Plan

ASSESSMENT Subjective Objective	Nursing diagnosis	GOALS Short-term Long-term	Implementation	Evaluation

Summary/Conclusion

Health Education

Reference

Date of submission: Signature of subject In-charge

CASE PRESENTATION

■ HISTORY TAKING AND PHYSICAL EXAMINATION AND NURSING

Nursing History

Name of the ward: ________________________ Student name: ____________________

Period from: ______________to ____________ Name of the hospital: ________________

Demographic Data

Name of the patient:	IP No:
Age:	Gender:
Marital status:	Nationality:
Language spoken:	Religion:
Occupation:	Education:
Income:	Address:
Date of admission:	Treatment received on arrival to hospital:
Provisional diagnosis:	Treatment received by patient on arrival:

History of Present Illness

Ask any or all of the following as appropriate and write a summary

Reason for visit: ____

When did the symptoms started: ____________________________________

General state of health: ____

Was the onset sudden or gradual: __________________________________

How often the problem occurs: _____________________________________

Has the problem occur before: _____________________________________

Treatment received on arrival to hospital: ___________________________

Chief Complaint

Eliciting a client's history not only assists with individualizing the plan of care but also help to establish a bond with that client.

Gather specific information regarding:

Onset:____.

Location:____.

Duration: ____.

Aggravating factors: ____.

Relieving factors: ____.

Associated manifestation: ____.

Past surgical history: ____.

Past medical history: ____.

Allergies: ____.

Medication History

Medication prescribed. Use of antihypertensive/diuretics/vasodilator/nitroglycerin/anticoagulant/dioxin/bronchodilators/contraceptive/hormones/steroids/antidepressant/psychotropic/thyroid hormones/over the counter medication/herbs note time and dosage and how often they are taking.

____

____

____

Allergies: Note and describe any environmental, food or drug allergies

____

Family History

Type of family: Nuclear/Joint family

Family Composition

Sl. No.	Name	Relationship to the patient	Age	Sex	Education	Occupation	Health status

Family Tree

Family History of Illness

Is there any family history of: Asthma/cancer/diabetes/epilepsy/hypertension/heart disease/hepatitis/hemophilia/ stroke/tuberculosis/mental disorders/thyroid or autoimmune disorders/aged grandparent and siblings alive? If yes, what is their current state of health? If no, state the cause of death and age of death ___________________________

____

Past Health History

- Previous hospitalization: ____

- Surgery if any: ____

- History of accident or blood transfusion: _______________________________

- Is the client taking any prescription or over-the-counter medications on a regular basis/notice all the medications, how long:____

Values and Beliefs

- What are the client's attitudes/beliefs about hospitalization?

____

- Does he/she have any inappropriate perception of illness?

____

Dietary Habits

Assess excess or deficit caloric intake and client approximate intake of foods, high in sodium, cholesterol, saturated fat, and caffeine.

____

____

■ PHYSICAL EXAMINATION

Use questioning, observation and examination to gather data. Tick items that apply to the client and comment as needed.

Sensation

Eyes:
- Poor vision/blurred vision/eye infection:
- Blindness R/L/eye pain:
- Itching/prosthesis/glasses/contact lens:

Ears: Ringing in ears/discharge/ear infection/loss of hearing R/L/ear pain/itching/hearing aids.

Tongue: Difficulty of taste.

Nose: Frequent colds/nose bleeds/pain/discharge.

Touch: Reduced or tactile perception.

Skin and mucus membranes: Excessive dryness/bruising/jaundice/itching/rash/broken skin/wound/pale/flushed/poor turgor/change in pigmentation.

Mouth and throat: Sore throat/coated tongue/dental caries/bad breath (halitosis)/bleeding gums/dentures upper/lower.

Hair: Itchy scalp/hygiene poor/dandruff/hair change/loss/excess.

Nails: Colors changes/biting/splitting/clubbing

Respiration

- Rate: _______________________________________
- Cough/dyspnea/wheezing/coughs blood (hemoptysis)/cyanosis/pain on breathing/restlessness—smoke (how many per day): _______________________________________

Circulation

- Pulse rate: _______________________________/min
- Blood pressure: _______________________________mm Hg
- Fatigue/Chest pain/nausea—vomiting/anemia/varicose veins/peripheral pulses/leg swelling/ulcers.

Nutrition

- Weight: _______________________________________
- Height: _______________________________________
- Skin fold thickness: _______________________________
- Appetite change/weight change/nausea/vomiting/dysphasia/heart burn/dentures/normal eating pattern (likes and dislikes):_______________________________

Abdomen

- **Inspection:** Rashes/lesions/scar/striae
- **Distended peristalsis:** Present/absent
- **Palpation:** Pain/tenderness/mass

Elimination

Urinary/frequency/urgency/dribbling/urinary incontinence/painful urination retention/dysuria/urinary appliance/nocturia/hematuria/anuria/distended bladder

Activity/Exercise

Muscle Pain/muscle weakness/cramps/joint pain/swelling/stiffness of movements/deformities/abnormal gait/fatigue/impaired coordination

Self-care (describe limitation to eating, bathing, dressing, toileting, ambulating) ______________________

____

Comfort

Describes the following:

Pain? If yes, how it is relieved?: ____

Sleep pattern and methods/treatment used for sleep: ________________________________

Neurological Responses

Disorientation/unconscious/headache/tremors/paralysis numbness/weakness/seizures (fits)/dizziness/loss of memory/difficult expressing self verbally.

Immune Response

- Temperature: _______________________________
- Allergies: _______________________________
- Fever in last 45 hours: _______________________________
- Swollen glands: _______________________________
- COMMENTS: _______________________________

Sexuality

Female:
- Age of menarche: _______________________________
- LMP: _______________________________
- Duration: _______________________________
- Flow: _______________________________
- Cycle: _______________________ days)/dysmenorrheal/bleeding between periods/vaginal bleeding.

Male:

Discharge/swelling/masses; comments: _______________________________

Comparing Theory Knowledge with Present Patient Condition

Knowledge of disease	As per theory knowledge	Present in patient
Definition		
Review related anatomy and physiology		

Knowledge of disease	As per theory knowledge	Present in patient
Etiology		
Diagnosis		
Clinical manifestation		
Diagnosis evaluation/investigation		
Medical management		
Surgical management		
Dietary management		

Nursing Care Plan

ASSESSMENT Subjective Objective	Nursing diagnosis	GOALS Short-term Long-term	Implementation	Evaluation

Summary/Conclusion

Health Education

Reference

Date of submission: **Signature of subject In-charge**

DRUG STUDY

Name of the Patient: _________________________ **Diagnosis:** _________________________

Name of the drug	Route of administration	Dosage and frequency	Indication	Contraindication	Adverse reaction	Nursing intervention

Date of submission:

Signature of subject supervisor:

SURGICAL WARD

NURSING CARE PLAN: 1

■ HISTORY TAKING AND PHYSICAL EXAMINATION

Nursing History

Name of the ward: ___________________________ Student name: ___________________________

Period from: _______________ to _______________ Name of the hospital: ___________________________

Demographic Data

Name of the patient:	IP No:
Age:	Gender:
Marital status:	Nationality:
Language spoken:	Religion:
Occupation:	Education:
Income:	Address:
Date of admission:	Treatment received on arrival to hospital:
Provisional diagnosis:	Treatment received by patient on arrival:

History of Present Illness

Ask any or all of the following as appropriate and write a summary

Reason for visit: ___________________________

When did the symptoms started: ___________________________

General state of health: ___________________________

Was the onset sudden or gradual: ___________________________

How often the problem occurs: ___________________________

Has the problem occur before: ___________________________

Treatment received on arrival to hospital: ___________________________

Chief Complaint

Eliciting a client's history not only assists with individualizing the plan of care but also help to establish a bond with that client.

Gather specific information regarding:

Onset: ___________________________.

Location: ___________________________.

Duration: ___________________________.

Aggravating factors: ___________________________.

Relieving factors: ___________________________.

Associated manifestation: ____ .

Past surgical history: ____ .

Past medical history: ____ .

Allergies: ____ .

Medication History

Medication prescribed. Use of antihypertensive/diuretics/vasodilator/nitroglycerin/anticoagulant/dioxin/bronchodilators/contraceptive/hormones/steroids/antidepressant/psychotropic/thyroid hormones/over the counter medication/herbs note time and dosage and how often they are taking.

____ .

____

____

Allergies: Note and describe any environmental, food or drug allergies

____

Family History

Type of family: Nuclear/Joint family

Family Composition

Sl. No.	Name	Relationship to the patient	Age	Sex	Education	Occupation	Health status

Family Tree

Family History of Illness
Is there any family history of: Asthma/cancer/diabetes/epilepsy/hypertension/heart disease/hepatitis/hemophilia/ stroke/tuberculosis/mental disorders/thyroid or autoimmune disorders/aged grandparent and siblings alive? If yes, what is their current state of health? If no, state the cause of death and age of death _______________________

____

Past Health History

- Previous hospitalization: ____

- Surgery if any: ____

- History of accident or blood transfusion: ____

- Is the client taking any prescription or over-the-counter medications on a regular basis/notice all the medications, how long: ____

____

Values and Beliefs

- What are the client's attitudes/beliefs about hospitalization?

____

- Does he/she have any inappropriate perception of illness?

____

Dietary Habits

Assess excess or deficit caloric intake and client approximate intake of foods, high in sodium, cholesterol, saturated fat, and caffeine.

____

____

■ PHYSICAL EXAMINATION

Use questioning, observation and examination to gather data. Tick items that apply to the client and comment as needed.

Sensation

Eyes:
- Poor vision/blurred vision/eye infection:
- Blindness R/L/eye pain:
- Itching/prosthesis/glasses/contact lens:

Ears: Ringing in ears/discharge/ear infection/loss of hearing R/L/ear pain/itching/hearing aids.

Tongue: Difficulty of taste.

Nose: Frequent colds/nose bleeds/pain/discharge.

Touch: Reduced or tactile perception.

Skin and mucus membranes: Excessive dryness/bruising/jaundice/itching/rash/broken skin/wound/pale/flushed/poor turgor/change in pigmentation.

Mouth and throat: Sore throat/coated tongue/dental caries/bad breath (halitosis)/bleeding gums/dentures upper/lower.

Hair: Itchy scalp/hygiene poor/dandruff/hair change/loss/excess.

Nails: Colors changes/biting/splitting/clubbing

Respiration

- Rate: _______________________________________
- Cough/dyspnea/wheezing/coughs blood (hemoptysis)/cyanosis/pain on breathing/restlessness—smoke (how many per day): _______________________________________

Circulation

- Pulse rate: _____________________________________/min
- Blood pressure: _______________________________mm Hg
- Fatigue/Chest pain/nausea—vomiting/anemia/varicose veins/peripheral pulses/leg swelling/ulcers.

Nutrition

- Weight: _______________________________________
- Height: _______________________________________
- Skin fold thickness: _______________________________
- Appetite change/weight change/nausea/vomiting/dysphasia/heart burn/dentures/normal eating pattern (likes and dislikes):_______________________________________

Abdomen

- **Inspection:** Rashes/lesions/scar/striae
- **Distended peristalsis:** Present/absent
- **Palpation:** Pain/tenderness/mass

Elimination

Urinary/frequency/urgency/dribbling/urinary incontinence/painful urination retention/dysuria/urinary appliance/nocturia/hematuria/anuria/distended bladder

Activity/Exercise

Muscle Pain/muscle weakness/cramps/joint pain/swelling/stiffness of movements/deformities/abnormal gait/fatigue/ impaired coordination

Self-care (describe limitation to eating, bathing, dressing, toileting, ambulating) ________________________

____

Comfort

Describes the following:

Pain? If yes, how it is relieved?: ____

Sleep pattern and methods/treatment used for sleep: ________________________________

Neurological Responses

Disorientation/unconscious/headache/tremors/paralysis numbness/weakness/seizures (fits)/dizziness/loss of memory/ difficult expressing self verbally.

Immune Response

- Temperature: ____
- Allergies: ____
- Fever in last 45 hours: ________________________________
- Swollen glands: _______________________________________
- COMMENTS:____

Sexuality

Female:
- Age of menarche: ______________________________________
- LMP: ____
- Duration: ____
- Flow: ____
- Cycle: ____________________________ days)/dysmenorrheal/bleeding between periods/vaginal bleeding.

Male:
Discharge/swelling/masses; comments: ____

Investigation Done

Date	Name of the investigation	Normal values	Patients values/result	Significance

Medical diagnosis (Final): ____

Surgical diagnosis: ____

Drug Management

Name of the drug	Dosage and frequency	Side effect	Nursing intervention

Diet Plan

Type of diet required (snacks, lunch, dinner):

____

____

____

____

____

____

____

____

____

____

____

Nursing Care Plan

ASSESSMENT Subjective Objective	Nursing diagnosis	GOALS Short-term Long-term	Implementation	Evaluation

Summary/Conclusion

Health Education

Reference

Date of submission: **Signature of subject In-charge:**

NURSING CARE PLAN: 2

■ HISTORY TAKING AND PHYSICAL EXAMINATION

Nursing History

Name of the ward: _________________________ Student name: _________________________

Period from: _______________to _______________ Name of the hospital: _________________________

Demographic Data

Name of the patient:	IP No:
Age:	Gender:
Marital status:	Nationality:
Language spoken:	Religion:
Occupation:	Education:
Income:	Address:
Date of admission:	Treatment received on arrival to hospital:
Provisional diagnosis:	Treatment received by patient on arrival:

History of Present Illness

Ask any or all of the following as appropriate and write a summary

Reason for visit: _________________________

When did the symptoms started: _________________________

General state of health: _________________________

Was the onset sudden or gradual: _________________________

How often the problem occurs: _________________________

Has the problem occur before: _________________________

Treatment received on arrival to hospital: _________________________

Chief Complaint

Eliciting a client's history not only assists with individualizing the plan of care but also help to establish a bond with that client.

Gather specific information regarding:

Onset:_________________________.

Location: _________________________.

Duration: _________________________.

Aggravating factors: _________________________.

Relieving factors: _________________________.

Associated manifestation: ____.

Past surgical history: ____.

Past medical history: ____.

Allergies: ____.

Medication History

Medication prescribed. Use of antihypertensive/diuretics/vasodilator/nitroglycerin/anticoagulant/dioxin/bronchodilators/contraceptive/hormones/steroids/antidepressant/psychotropic/thyroid hormones/over the counter medication/herbs note time and dosage and how often they are taking.

____

____

____

Allergies: Note and describe any environmental, food or drug allergies

____

Family History

Type of family: Nuclear/Joint family

Family Composition

Sl. No.	Name	Relationship to the patient	Age	Sex	Education	Occupation	Health status

Family Tree

Family History of Illness

Is there any family history of: Asthma/cancer/diabetes/epilepsy/hypertension/heart disease/hepatitis/hemophilia/stroke/tuberculosis/mental disorders/thyroid or autoimmune disorders/aged grandparent and siblings alive? If yes, what is their current state of health? If no, state the cause of death and age of death ______________

____

Past Health History

- Previous hospitalization: ____
- Surgery if any: ____
- History of accident or blood transfusion: ______________________________
- Is the client taking any prescription or over-the-counter medications on a regular basis/notice all the medications, how long: ______________________________________

Values and Beliefs

- What are the client's attitudes/beliefs about hospitalization?

____

- Does he/she have any inappropriate perception of illness?

____

Dietary Habits

Assess excess or deficit caloric intake and client approximate intake of foods, high in sodium, cholesterol, saturated fat, and caffeine.

____

____

▉ PHYSICAL EXAMINATION

Use questioning, observation and examination to gather data. Tick items that apply to the client and comment as needed.

Sensation

Eyes:
- Poor vision/blurred vision/eye infection:
- Blindness R/L/eye pain:
- Itching/prosthesis/glasses/contact lens:

Ears: Ringing in ears/discharge/ear infection/loss of hearing R/L/ear pain/itching/hearing aids.

Tongue: Difficulty of taste.

Nose: Frequent colds/nose bleeds/pain/discharge.

Touch: Reduced or tactile perception.

Skin and mucus membranes: Excessive dryness/bruising/jaundice/itching/rash/broken skin/wound/pale/flushed/poor turgor/change in pigmentation.

Mouth and throat: Sore throat/coated tongue/dental caries/bad breath (halitosis)/bleeding gums/dentures upper/lower.

Hair: Itchy scalp/hygiene poor/dandruff/hair change/loss/excess.

Nails: Colors changes/biting/splitting/clubbing

Respiration

- Rate: _______________________________
- Cough/dyspnea/wheezing/coughs blood (hemoptysis)/cyanosis/pain on breathing/restlessness—smoke (how many per day): _______________________________

Circulation

- Pulse rate: _______________________________/min
- Blood pressure: _______________________________mm Hg
- Fatigue/Chest pain/nausea—vomiting/anemia/varicose veins/peripheral pulses/leg swelling/ulcers.

Nutrition

- Weight: _______________________________
- Height: _______________________________
- Skin fold thickness: _______________________________
- Appetite change/weight change/nausea/vomiting/dysphasia/heart burn/dentures/normal eating pattern (likes and dislikes): _______________________________

Abdomen

- **Inspection:** Rashes/lesions/scar/striae
- **Distended peristalsis:** Present/absent
- **Palpation:** Pain/tenderness/mass

Elimination

Urinary/frequency/urgency/dribbling/urinary incontinence/painful urination retention/dysuria/urinary appliance/nocturia/hematuria/anuria/distended bladder

Activity/Exercise

Muscle Pain/muscle weakness/cramps/joint pain/swelling/stiffness of movements/deformities/abnormal gait/fatigue/impaired coordination

Self-care (describe limitation to eating, bathing, dressing, toileting, ambulating) _______________________

____

Comfort

Describes the following:

Pain? If yes, how it is relieved?: _______________________

Sleep pattern and methods/treatment used for sleep: _______________________

Neurological Responses

Disorientation/unconscious/headache/tremors/paralysis numbness/weakness/seizures (fits)/dizziness/loss of memory/difficult expressing self verbally.

Immune Response

- Temperature: _______________________
- Allergies: _______________________
- Fever in last 45 hours: _______________________
- Swollen glands: _______________________
- COMMENTS: _______________________

Sexuality

Female:
- Age of menarche: _______________________
- LMP: _______________________
- Duration: _______________________
- Flow: _______________________
- Cycle: _______________________ days)/dysmenorrheal/bleeding between periods/vaginal bleeding.

Male:

Discharge/swelling/masses; comments: _______________________

Investigation Done

Date	Name of the investigation	Normal values	Patients values/result	Significance

Medical diagnosis (Final): _______________________

Surgical diagnosis: _______________________

Drug Management

Name of the drug	Dosage and frequency	Side effect	Nursing intervention

Diet Plan

Type of diet required (snacks, lunch, dinner):

____

____

____

____

____

____

____

____

____

____

____

Nursing Care Plan

ASSESSMENT Subjective Objective	Nursing diagnosis	GOALS Short-term Long-term	Implementation	Evaluation

Summary/Conclusion

Health Education

Reference

Date of submission: **Signature of subject In-charge:**

CASE STUDY

■ HISTORY TAKING AND PHYSICAL EXAMINATION

Nursing History

Name of the ward: _______________________ Student name: _______________________

Period from: _______________to _______________ Name of the hospital: _______________________

Demographic Data

Name of the patient:	IP No:
Age:	Gender:
Marital status:	Nationality:
Language spoken:	Religion:
Occupation:	Education:
Income:	Address:
Date of admission:	Treatment received on arrival to hospital:
Provisional diagnosis:	Treatment received by patient on arrival:

History of Present Illness

Ask any or all of the following as appropriate and write a summary

Reason for visit: _______________________

When did the symptoms started: _______________________

General state of health: _______________________

Was the onset sudden or gradual: _______________________

How often the problem occurs: _______________________

Has the problem occur before: _______________________

Treatment received on arrival to hospital: _______________________

Chief Complaint

Eliciting a client's history not only assists with individualizing the plan of care but also help to establish a bond with that client.

Gather specific information regarding:

Onset: _______________________

Location: _______________________

Duration: _______________________

Aggravating factors: _______________________

Relieving factors: _______________________

Associated manifestation: ____.

Past surgical history: ____.

Past medical history: ____.

Allergies: ____.

Medication History

Medication prescribed. Use of antihypertensive/diuretics/vasodilator/nitroglycerin/anticoagulant/dioxin/bronchodilators/contraceptive/hormones/steroids/antidepressant/psychotropic/thyroid hormones/over the counter medication/herbs note time and dosage and how often they are taking.

____

____

____

Allergies: Note and describe any environmental, food or drug allergies

____

Family History

Type of family: Nuclear/Joint family

Family Composition

Sl. No.	Name	Relationship to the patient	Age	Sex	Education	Occupation	Health status

Family Tree

Family History of Illness

Is there any family history of: Asthma/cancer/diabetes/epilepsy/hypertension/heart disease/hepatitis/hemophilia/ stroke/tuberculosis/mental disorders/thyroid or autoimmune disorders/aged grandparent and siblings alive? If yes, what is their current state of health? If no, state the cause of death and age of death _______________________

____

Past Health History

- Previous hospitalization: ____

- Surgery if any: ____

- History of accident or blood transfusion: ____

- Is the client taking any prescription or over-the-counter medications on a regular basis/notice all the medications, how long: ____

____

Values and Beliefs

- What are the client's attitudes/beliefs about hospitalization?

____

- Does he/she have any inappropriate perception of illness?

____

Dietary Habits

Assess excess or deficit caloric intake and client approximate intake of foods, high in sodium, cholesterol, saturated fat, and caffeine.

____

____

■ PHYSICAL EXAMINATION

Use questioning, observation and examination to gather data. Tick items that apply to the client and comment as needed.

Sensation

Eyes:
- Poor vision/blurred vision/eye infection:
- Blindness R/L/eye pain:
- Itching/prosthesis/glasses/contact lens:

Ears: Ringing in ears/discharge/ear infection/loss of hearing R/L/ear pain/itching/hearing aids.

Tongue: Difficulty of taste.

Nose: Frequent colds/nose bleeds/pain/discharge.

Touch: Reduced or tactile perception.

Skin and mucus membranes: Excessive dryness/bruising/jaundice/itching/rash/broken skin/wound/pale/flushed/poor turgor/change in pigmentation.

Mouth and throat: Sore throat/coated tongue/dental caries/bad breath (halitosis)/bleeding gums/dentures upper/lower.

Hair: Itchy scalp/hygiene poor/dandruff/hair change/loss/excess.

Nails: Colors changes/biting/splitting/clubbing

Respiration

- Rate: ____
- Cough/dyspnea/wheezing/coughs blood (hemoptysis)/cyanosis/pain on breathing/restlessness—smoke (how many per day): ____

Circulation

- Pulse rate: ____/min
- Blood pressure: ___________________________________mm Hg
- Fatigue/Chest pain/nausea—vomiting/anemia/varicose veins/peripheral pulses/leg swelling/ulcers.

Nutrition

- Weight: _______________________________________
- Height: _______________________________________
- Skin fold thic   kness: _______________________________
- Appetite change/weight change/nausea/vomiting/dysphasia/heart burn/dentures/normal eating pattern (likes and dislikes): _______________________________________

Abdomen

- **Inspection:** Rashes/lesions/scar/striae
- **Distended peristalsis:** Present/absent
- **Palpation:** Pain/tenderness/mass

Elimination

Urinary/frequency/urgency/dribbling/urinary incontinence/painful urination retention/dysuria/urinary appliance/nocturia/hematuria/anuria/distended bladder

Activity/Exercise

Muscle Pain/muscle weakness/cramps/joint pain/swelling/stiffness of movements/deformities/abnormal gait/fatigue/impaired coordination

Self-care (describe limitation to eating, bathing, dressing, toileting, ambulating) _______________________

____

Comfort

Describes the following:

Pain? If yes, how it is relieved?: ____

Sleep pattern and methods/treatment used for sleep: _______________________________

Neurological Responses

Disorientation/unconscious/headache/tremors/paralysis numbness/weakness/seizures (fits)/dizziness/loss of memory/difficult expressing self verbally.

Immune Response

- Temperature: _______________________________
- Allergies: _________________________________
- Fever in last 45 hours: _____________________
- Swollen glands: ____________________________
- COMMENTS:________________________________

Sexuality

Female:
- Age of menarche: ___________________________
- LMP: _____________________________________
- Duration: _________________________________
- Flow: _____________________________________
- Cycle: _______________________ days)/dysmenorrheal/bleeding between periods/vaginal bleeding.

Male:

Discharge/swelling/masses; comments: ____

Comparing Theory Knowledge with Present Patient Condition

Knowledge of disease	As per theory knowledge	Present in patient
Definition		
Review related anatomy and physiology		

Knowledge of disease	As per theory knowledge	Present in patient
Etiology		
Diagnosis		
Clinical manifestation		
Diagnosis evaluation/ investigation		
Medical management		
Surgical management		
Dietary management		

Nursing Care Plan

ASSESSMENT Subjective Objective	Nursing diagnosis	GOALS Short-term Long-term	Implementation	Evaluation

Summary/Conclusion

Health Education

Reference

Date of submission: **Signature of subject In-charge:**

CASE PRESENTATION

■ HISTORY TAKING AND PHYSICAL EXAMINATION

Nursing History

Name of the ward: _________________________ Student name: _____________________

Period from: _______________ to _______________ Name of the hospital: _________________

Demographic Data

Name of the patient:	IP No:
Age:	Gender:
Marital status:	Nationality:
Language spoken:	Religion:
Occupation:	Education:
Income:	Address:
Date of admission:	Treatment received on arrival to hospital:
Provisional diagnosis:	Treatment received by patient on arrival:

History of Present Illness

Ask any or all of the following as appropriate and write a summary

Reason for visit: ____

When did the symptoms started: ____

General state of health: ____

Was the onset sudden or gradual: ____

How often the problem occurs: ____

Has the problem occur before: ____

Treatment received on arrival to hospital: ____

Chief Complaint

Eliciting a client's history not only assists with individualizing the plan of care but also help to establish a bond with that client.

Gather specific information regarding:

Onset: ____.

Location: ____.

Duration: ____.

Aggravating factors: ____.

Relieving factors: ____.

Associated manifestation: ____.

Past surgical history: ____.

Past medical history: ____.

Allergies: ____.

Medication History

Medication prescribed. Use of antihypertensive/diuretics/vasodilator/nitroglycerin/anticoagulant/dioxin/bronchodilators/contraceptive/hormones/steroids/antidepressant/psychotropic/thyroid hormones/over the counter medication/herbs note time and dosage and how often they are taking.

____

____

____

Allergies: Note and describe any environmental, food or drug allergies

____

Family History

Type of family: Nuclear/Joint family

Family Composition

Sl. No.	Name	Relationship to the patient	Age	Sex	Education	Occupation	Health status

Family Tree

Family History of Illness

Is there any family history of: Asthma/cancer/diabetes/epilepsy/hypertension/heart disease/hepatitis/hemophilia/stroke/tuberculosis/mental disorders/thyroid or autoimmune disorders/aged grandparent and siblings alive? If yes, what is their current state of health? If no, state the cause of death and age of death ________________________

____

Past Health History

- Previous hospitalization: ____

- Surgery if any: ____

- History of accident or blood transfusion: ________________________________

- Is the client taking any prescription or over-the-counter medications on a regular basis/notice all the medications, how long: ________________________________

Values and Beliefs

- What are the client's attitudes/beliefs about hospitalization?

____

- Does he/she have any inappropriate perception of illness?

____

Dietary Habits

Assess excess or deficit caloric intake and client approximate intake of foods, high in sodium, cholesterol, saturated fat, and caffeine.

____

____

■ PHYSICAL EXAMINATION

Use questioning, observation and examination to gather data. Tick items that apply to the client and comment as needed.

Sensation

Eyes:
- Poor vision/blurred vision/eye infection:
- Blindness R/L/eye pain:
- Itching/prosthesis/glasses/contact lens:

Ears: Ringing in ears/discharge/ear infection/loss of hearing R/L/ear pain/itching/hearing aids.

Tongue: Difficulty of taste.

Nose: Frequent colds/nose bleeds/pain/discharge.

Touch: Reduced or tactile perception.

Skin and mucus membranes: Excessive dryness/bruising/jaundice/itching/rash/broken skin/wound/pale/flushed/poor turgor/change in pigmentation.

Mouth and throat: Sore throat/coated tongue/dental caries/bad breath (halitosis)/bleeding gums/dentures upper/lower.

Hair: Itchy scalp/hygiene poor/dandruff/hair change/loss/excess.

Nails: Colors changes/biting/splitting/clubbing

Respiration

- Rate: ____
- Cough/dyspnea/wheezing/coughs blood (hemoptysis)/cyanosis/pain on breathing/restlessness—smoke (how many per day): ____

Circulation

- Pulse rate: ____/min
- Blood pressure: _________________________________mm Hg
- Fatigue/Chest pain/nausea—vomiting/anemia/varicose veins/peripheral pulses/leg swelling/ulcers.

Nutrition

- Weight: _______________________________________
- Height: _______________________________________
- Skin fold thickness: ___________________________
- Appetite change/weight change/nausea/vomiting/dysphasia/heart burn/dentures/normal eating pattern (likes and dislikes):____

Abdomen

- **Inspection:** Rashes/lesions/scar/striae
- **Distended peristalsis:** Present/absent
- **Palpation:** Pain/tenderness/mass

Elimination

Urinary/frequency/urgency/dribbling/urinary incontinence/painful urination retention/dysuria/urinary appliance/nocturia/hematuria/anuria/distended bladder

Activity/Exercise

Muscle Pain/muscle weakness/cramps/joint pain/swelling/stiffness of movements/deformities/abnormal gait/fatigue/impaired coordination

Self-care (describe limitation to eating, bathing, dressing, toileting, ambulating) _______________________

____

Comfort

Describes the following:

Pain? If yes, how it is relieved?: ____

Sleep pattern and methods/treatment used for sleep: ________________________________

Neurological Responses

Disorientation/unconscious/headache/tremors/paralysis numbness/weakness/seizures (fits)/dizziness/loss of memory/difficult expressing self verbally.

Immune Response

- Temperature: _______________________________
- Allergies: _______________________________
- Fever in last 45 hours: _______________________________
- Swollen glands: _______________________________
- COMMENTS: _______________________________

Sexuality

Female:
- Age of menarche: _______________________________
- LMP: _______________________________
- Duration: _______________________________
- Flow: _______________________________
- Cycle: _______________________ days)/dysmenorrheal/bleeding between periods/vaginal bleeding.

Male:

Discharge/swelling/masses; comments: _______________________________

Comparing Theory Knowledge with Present Patient Condition

Knowledge of disease	As per theory knowledge	Present in patient
Definition		
Review related anatomy and physiology		

Knowledge of disease	As per theory knowledge	Present in patient
Etiology		
Diagnosis		
Clinical manifestation		
Diagnosis evaluation/ investigation		
Medical management		
Surgical management		
Dietary management		

Nursing Care Plan

ASSESSMENT Subjective Objective	Nursing diagnosis	GOALS Short-term Long-term	Implementation	Evaluation

Summary/Conclusion

Health Education

Reference

Date of submission:

Signature of subject In-charge:

DRUG STUDY

Name of the Patient: _________________________ **Diagnosis:** _________________________

Name of the drug	Route of administration	Dosage and frequency	Indication	Contraindication	Adverse reaction	Nursing intervention

Date of submission: **Signature of subject supervisor:**

OBSERVATION REPORT ON SURGICAL OPD

Date of submission: **Signature of subject In-charge:**

OBSERVATION REPORT IN OPERATION THEATER

Date of submission: Signature of subject In-charge:

OBSERVATION REPORT IN ORTHOPEDIC WARD

Date of submission:

Signature of subject In-charge:

OBSERVATION REPORT IN ICU

Date of submission:

Signature of subject In-charge:

OBSERVATION REPORT ON CASUALTY/EMERGENCY

Date of submission: **Signature of subject In-charge:**

INTAKE AND OUTPUT CHART

Name of the patient _______________________________ **IP No.** _______________________

Diagnosis _______________________________ **Date of admission** _______________________

Intake					Output			
Date	Time	RT	Parenteral route	Oral	Urine	Drainage/ suction/ aspirated	Vomitus Diarrhea	Total

Total intake for 24 hours _______________________________

Total output for 24 hours _______________________________

Signature of submission: **Signature of Subject In-charge:**

MEDICAL GADGET/DEVICES

Performa for Medical Gadget/Device Presentation

Name of the ward _________________________ Name of the teacher _________________________

Sl. No.	Name of the device	Device maintenance	Function of the device
1.			
2.			
3.			
4.			
5.			
6.			
7.			
8.			
9.			
10.			

Evaluation of gadget ____

Date of submission: Signature of subject In-charge:

NEW LEARNING

New Learning: Date ________________________ Name of the Area ________________________

Date	New technique/procedure	Nursing role

New Learning: Date ________________________ Name of the Area ________________________

Date	New technique/procedure	Nursing role

New Learning: Date ________________________ Name of the Area ________________________

Date	New technique/procedure	Nursing role

New Learning: Date ________________________ Name of the Area ________________________

Date	New technique/procedure	Nursing role

MEDICAL SURGICAL NURSING CLINICAL ASSESSMENT

Performance Evaluation

Student name ____

Medical surgical unit ___________________ Ward ________________ From _____________ to _____________

Date ____

■ PERFORMANCE CRITERIA

Sl. No.	Standard	SM (4 M)	SAM (3M)	SAM (2M)	SNM (1M)
	Nursing Knowledge				
	Assessment and Nursing Diagnosis				
1.	Collect thorough knowledge about patient illness				
2.	Recognizes the physical needs of the patient				
3.	Identifies psychological needs of the patient and family				
4.	Categorizes the patient problems				
5.	Formulates complete nursing diagnosis				
	Planning				
6.	Prioritizes the patient needs				
7.	Establishes suitable nursing actions for each patient's needs				
8.	Competent in implementing nursing care thorough, safe and accurate, collects and replaces equipment, organizes activities within time				
9.	Maintains comfortable environment for patient				
10.	Maintains safe therapeutic environment				
11.	Accurately records and reports patient information				
12.	Able to give planned health instructions to patient and family				
	Evaluation				
13.	Establishes outcome criteria for the patient including physical state, behavior and response to				
14.	Rationale able to state rationale for nursing actions				
	Medical Knowledge				
15.	Drug file presents written document as follows: Name of the drug, action, indications, dosage, ranges, contraindications, side effects, precautions.				

16.	Medical diagnosis: States accurate medical diagnosis) of each patient cared for and describes etiology, signs and symptoms, medical therapy and results of medical therapy				
17.	Laboratory investigation: States proper names of laboratory investigations of each patient cared for and describe reasons for tests, patient preparation for tests, test procedure				
Professional Conduct					
18.	Uniform: Always well groomed and neat, conscious about professional appearance				
19.	Punctuality: Exceptionally punctual for clinical and has never been late, completes all learning assignments on time				
20.	Sense of Responsibility: Readily accepts responsibility, reliable, adaptable and displays consistency in work, judgment is consistently sound and logical, works effectively under pressure				
21.	Initiative for self-learning: Eager to learn and seek new learning experiences self-directives in expanding knowledge and utilizing available resources and has original ideas.				
Communication Skill					
22.	Patient and family: Establishes and maintains outstanding working relationships with patients and families				
23.	Hospital staff/health team: Establishes harmonious relationship with the members of the health team, deals with them skillfully, smoothly and with insight. Polite and helpful				
24.	Colleagues: Very well accepted by colleagues. Always concerned about them and works well with them				
25.	Teachers: Always respects rules and regulations, accepts constructive criticism				

(SM: standard met; SAM: standard almost met; SFFM: standard average met; SNM: standard not met completely).

Total marks _________________________ **Total marks obtained** _______________________

Signature of teacher ____

PSYCHIATRIC WARD

NURSING CARE PLAN FOR PATIENT WITH PSYCHIATRIC DISORDERS

■ HISTORY TAKING AND MENTAL STATUS EXAMINATION

Identification Data

Name	Age
Sex	Father/spouse
Education	Occupation
Income	Marital status
Religion	IP Number
Diagnosis	Address _______________________ _______________________ Informant:
Treatment received on arrival to hospital _______________________________________ ____ ____	

History of Present Psychiatric Illness

What problem made you to come/bring to hospital?

____

When this symptoms started?

____

Any precipitating factors/aggravating factors?

____

Was the onset sudden or gradual?

____

How often does the problem occurs?

____

Has the problem occurs before?

____

Consider abnormal behavior, associated problem and disruptive behavior like suicide/homicide, changes in mood, thought, speech and abnormal perception _______________________________________

____

____

Reason for admission ____

Type of admission ____

Past Medical History

Any history of illness–hospitalization? If yes, history of diagnosis and treatment:

____

____

____

Any medical events, such as head injury, surgery, DM, hypertension, convulsion:

____

____

____

Past psychiatric illness (according to patient relatives):

____

____

____

____

____

____

____

____

____

History of hospitalization: Yes/No

Treatment taken: Yes/No

Psychological therapy: ____

____

____

Previous episode of any mental illness:

____

____

____

____

Family History of Psychiatric Illness

Sl. No.	Name of the family member	Age	Relationship with patient	Any psychiatric illness

Family Tree

Personal History

Perinatal history:
Antenatal period eventful/uneventful: ______________________________
Exposure to radiation/drug/infection: ______________________________
Natural birth, premature/normal/delivery/forceps delivery/caesarian section/instrumental delivery.
Birth cry: Immediate/delayed
Bonding: Immediate/delayed
Reaction of parents to childbirth: ______________________________
Separation from mother: Yes/No
Postnatal complications:
Under–weight/infection/separations/underweight/infection/delayed breastfeeding: ______________
Childhood history:
Parent relationship with the child: Harmonious/disturbed
Developmental milestone as per age: Normal/delayed
Relationship with family members: Normal/disturbed
Immunization received as per schedule: Yes/No
Feeding: Breastfeeding/artificial mode
Weaning: Response to weaning ______________________________
Behavior: Temper tantrum/thumb sucking/stuttering/head banging/nail biting/night mares.
Educational history:
Academic achievement: Normal/underachiever
Extracurricular activity: Normal/underachiever
Relationship with teacher: Good/disturbed

Attendance to school: Adequate/frequent absent

Relationship with peers: Normal/not adjusting

Attitude towards schooling: Positive/Negative

Reason for discontinuing study if any: _______________________________________

Play history:

Participate in games sports: Yes/No. If yes, like to play individual/with group.

Relationship with playmates: Good/not adjustable

Puberty:

Age at menarche ___________________________Reaction to menarche_________________

Regularity of cycle___________________________Duration of flow _________________

Occupational history:

Job started at what age: _______________________________________

Relationship with superior/colleagues/subordinate: Satisfactory/not satisfactory: ___________

Sexual and marital history:

Type of marriage _______________________________________

Duration of marriage_______________________________________

Relationship with spouse_______________________________________

Marital disharmony, if any: _______________________________________

Interest and hobbies:

Relationship with neighbors: _______________________________________

Hobbies: _______________________________________

Premorbid personality:

Predominant mood: Anxious/pessimistic/optimistic/stable/fluctuating.

Personality: Shy/suspicious/irritable/self–centered/impulsive/unconfidence/obsessional.

■ PHYSICAL EXAMINATION

Vital signs: Temperature ______________Pulse____________Respiration________________BP_____________

Any significant changes in CVS System: _______________________________________

Any significant changes in respiratory system: _______________________________________

Any significant changes in GI system: _______________________________________

Any significant changes in musculoskeletal system: _______________________________________

Any significant changes in reproductive system: _______________________________________

Any significant changes in integumentary system: _______________________________________

Any significant changes in respiratory system: _______________________________________

Any other medical problems: _______________________________________

■ MENTAL STATUS EXAMINATION

General Appearance

- **Level of grooming:** Normal/stability dressing/overdressed/idiosyncratically dressed.
- **Level of cleanliness:** Adequate/inadequate/overtly clean
- **Level of consciousness:** Fully conscious/alert/drowsy/stupors/comatose

- **Mode of hospital admission:** Came to hospital willingly/persuaded/brought using physical force
- **Cooperativeness:** Normal/more than so/less than so
- **Eye to eye contact:** Normal/increased/decreased
- **Psychomotor activity:** Normal/increased/decreased
- **Rapport:** Spontaneous/difficult/not to establish
- **Gesture:** Grimace/tics/mannerism
- **Posturing:** Stereotype/tremors/extrapyramidal
- **Other movement:** Stereotype/tremors/extrapyramidal
- **Other catatonic phenomena:** Automatic obedience/negativism/excessive cooperation/waxy flexibility/echopraxia/echolalia.
- **Conversion and disassociate sign:** Yes/no
- **Compulsive act or rituals:** Yes/no
- **Hallucinatory behavior:** Yes/no

Speech

- **Initiation:** Spontaneous/speak when spoken/minimal/mute
- **Reaction time:** Normal/delayed/shortened/difficulty
- **Rate:** Normal/delayed
- **Tone:** Normal variation/monotonous
- **Others:** Rhyming/echolalia/neologism

Mood and Affect

- **Mood:** Angry/hopeless/retarded/thought block/flight of ideas
- **Affect:** Appropriate to mood/blunt/flat. If inappropriate, explain patient expression

____

____

Thinking and Perception

- **Stream of thought:**
    - Pressure of thought: Unusually rapid/abundant/varied.
    - Poverty of thoughts: Unusually slow/few or unvaried thoughts.
    - Blocking of thoughts: Abrupt/complete emptying of mind.
- **Form of thought:** Associative looseness/flight of ideas/incoherent/perseveration
- **Thought content:** Preoccupations/morbid thoughts/obsession/compulsion/delusion
    If delusion present mention the type: _______________________________________
- **Perceptual disturbances:**
    - Hallucinations/illusions. If present, mention the type _______________________
    - Depersonalization/derealization

Orientation

- **Time:** Normal/impaired
- **Place:** Normal/impaired
- **Person:** Normal/impaired

Attention and Concentration

- **Attention:** Normal/Impaired
- **Concentration:** Normally sustained/sustained with difficulty

Memory

- **Immediate:** Intact/absent
- **Recent:** Intact/absent
- **Remote:** Intact/absent

Insight

- **Complete denial of illness:** Yes/No
- **Slight awareness of illness but in denial:** Yes/No
- **Awareness of illness but blaming others:** Yes/No
- **Intellectual insight:** Yes/No
- **True emotional insight:** Yes/No

Judgement

- **Personal judgment:** Intact/impaired
- **Social judgment:** Intact/impaired
- **Test judgment:** Intact/impaired

Investigation Done

Date	Name of the investigation	Normal values	Patients values/result	Significance

Diagnosis (Final) ____

Drug Management

Sl. No.	Name of the drug	Dosage and frequency	Route	Action	Side effect	Nursing intervention

Diet Plan

24 hours Nutritional Requirements

Type of diet required (snacks, lunch, dinner)

Time	Type	Quantity	Frequency	Remarks

List of Nursing Diagnosis/Problems/Need Identified According to Priority

1. ____
2. ____
3. ____
4. ____
5. ____

Nursing Care Plan

ASSESSMENT Subjective Objective	Nursing diagnosis	GOALS Short-term Long-term	Implementation	Evaluation

Summary/Conclusion

Health Education

Reference

Date of submission: **Signature of subject In-charge:**

CASE STUDY

■ HISTORY TAKING AND MENTAL STATUS EXAMINATION

Identification Data

Name	Age
Sex	Father/spouse
Education	Occupation
Income	Marital status
Religion	IP Number
Diagnosis	Address _______________________ Informant:
Treatment received on arrival to hospital ________________________ ____	

History of Present Psychiatric Illness

What problem made you to come/bring to hospital?

____

When this symptoms started?

____

Any precipitating factors/aggravating factors?

____

Was the onset sudden or gradual?

____

How often does the problem occurs?

____

Has the problem occurs before?

____

Consider abnormal behavior, associated problem and disruptive behavior like suicide/homicide, changes in mood , thought, speech and abnormal perception ________________________

____

____

Reason for admission ________________________

Type of admission ________________________

Past Medical History

Any history of illness–hospitalization? If yes, history of diagnosis and treatment:

____

____

____

____

Any medical events, such as head injury, surgery, DM, hypertension, convulsion:

____

____

____

____

Past psychiatric illness (according to patient relatives):

____

____

____

____

____

____

____

____

____

____

____

____

____

____

History of hospitalization: Yes/No

Treatment taken: Yes/No

Psychological therapy: ____

____

____

____

Previous episode of any mental illness:

____

____

____

____

Family History of Psychiatric Illness

Sl. No.	Name of the family member	Age	Relationship with patient	Any psychiatric illness

Family Tree

Personal History

Perinatal history:

Antenatal period eventful/uneventful: _______________________________

Exposure to radiation/drug/infection: _______________________________

Natural birth, premature/normal/delivery/forceps delivery/caesarian section/instrumental delivery.

Birth cry: Immediate/delayed

Bonding: Immediate/delayed

Reaction of parents to childbirth: _______________________________

Separation from mother: Yes/No

Postnatal complications:

Under-weight/infection/separations/underweight/infection/delayed breastfeeding: _______________________________

Childhood history:

Parent relationship with the child: Harmonious/disturbed

Developmental milestone as per age: Normal/delayed

Relationship with family members: Normal/disturbed

Immunization received as per schedule: Yes/No

Feeding: Breastfeeding/artificial mode

Weaning: Response to weaning _______________________________

Behavior: Temper tantrum/thumb sucking/stuttering/head banging/nail biting/night mares.

Educational history:

Academic achievement: Normal/underachiever

Extracurricular activity: Normal/underachiever

Relationship with teacher: Good/disturbed

Attendance to school: Adequate/frequent absent

Relationship with peers: Normal/not adjusting

Attitude towards schooling: Positive/Negative

Reason for discontinuing study if any: _______________________________

Play history:

Participate in games sports: Yes/No. If yes, like to play individual/with group.

Relationship with playmates: Good/not adjustable

Puberty:

Age at menarche _______________ Reaction to menarche _______________

Regularity of cycle _______________ Duration of flow _______________

Occupational history:

Job started at what age: _______________________________

Relationship with superior/colleagues/subordinate: Satisfactory/not satisfactory: _______________________________

Sexual and marital history:

Type of marriage ____

Duration of marriage____

Relationship with spouse____

Marital disharmony, if any: ____

Interest and hobbies:

Relationship with neighbors: ____

Hobbies: ____

Premorbid personality:

Predominant mood: Anxious/pessimistic/optimistic/stable/fluctuating.

Personality: Shy/suspicious/irritable/self–centered/impulsive/unconfidence/obsessional.

■ PHYSICAL EXAMINATION

Vital signs: Temperature ______________Pulse____________Respiration__________________BP__________________

Any significant changes in CVS System: _______________________________

Any significant changes in respiratory system: _______________________________

Any significant changes in GI system: _______________________________

Any significant changes in musculoskeletal system: _______________________________

Any significant changes in reproductive system: _______________________________

Any significant changes in integumentary system: _______________________________

Any significant changes in respiratory system: _______________________________

Any other medical problems: _______________________________

■ MENTAL STATUS EXAMINATION

General Appearance

- **Level of grooming:** Normal/stability dressing/overdressed/idiosyncratically dressed.
- **Level of cleanliness:** Adequate/inadequate/overtly clean
- **Level of consciousness:** Fully conscious/alert/drowsy/stupors/comatose
- **Mode of hospital admission:** Came to hospital willingly/persuaded/brought using physical force
- **Cooperativeness:** Normal/more than so/less than so
- **Eye to eye contact:** Normal/increased/decreased
- **Psychomotor activity:** Normal/increased/decreased
- **Rapport:** Spontaneous/difficult/not to establish
- **Gesture:** Grimace/tics/mannerism
- **Posturing:** Stereotype/tremors/extrapyramidal
- **Other movement:** Stereotype/tremors/extrapyramidal
- **Other catatonic phenomena:** Automatic obedience/negativism/excessive cooperation/waxy flexibility/echopraxia/echolalia.
- **Conversion and disassociate sign:** Yes/no
- **Compulsive act or rituals:** Yes/no
- **Hallucinatory behavior:** Yes/no

Speech

- **Initiation:** Spontaneous/speak when spoken/minimal/mute
- **Reaction time:** Normal/delayed/shortened/difficulty
- **Rate:** Normal/delayed
- **Tone:** Normal variation/monotonous
- **Others:** Rhyming/echolalia/neologism

Mood and Affect

- **Mood:** Angry/hopeless/retarded/thought block/flight of ideas
- **Affect:** Appropriate to mood/blunt/flat. If inappropriate, explain patient expression

____

____

Thinking and Perception

- **Stream of thought:**
    - Pressure of thought: Unusually rapid/abundant/varied.
    - Poverty of thoughts: Unusually slow/few or unvaried thoughts.
    - Blocking of thoughts: Abrupt/complete emptying of mind.
- **Form of thought:** Associative looseness/flight of ideas/incoherent/perseveration
- **Thought content:** Preoccupations/morbid thoughts/obsession/compulsion/delusion
  If delusion present mention the type: ____
- **Perceptual disturbances:**
    - Hallucinations/illusions. If present, mention the type _______________________________
    - Depersonalization/derealization

Orientation

- **Time:** Normal/impaired
- **Place:** Normal/impaired
- **Person:** Normal/impaired

Attention and Concentration

- **Attention:** Normal/Impaired
- **Concentration:** Normally sustained/sustained with difficulty

Memory

- **Immediate:** Intact/absent
- **Recent:** Intact/absent
- **Remote:** Intact/absent

Insight

- **Complete denial of illness:** Yes/No
- **Slight awareness of illness but in denial:** Yes/No
- **Awareness of illness but blaming others:** Yes/No
- **Intellectual insight:** Yes/No
- **True emotional insight:** Yes/No

Judgement

- **Personal judgment:** Intact/impaired
- **Social judgment:** Intact/impaired
- **Test judgment:** Intact/impaired

Book Picture and Patient Condition Comparison

Book picture	Patient condition
Etiology	
Psychopathology	
Clinical manifestation	
Investigation	
Diagnosis	
Psychopharmacology management	

Drug Study

Name of the drug	Dosage and frequency	Route	Action	Side effect	Nursing intervention

Diet Plan

24 hours Nutritional Requirements

Type of diet required (snacks, lunch, dinner)

Time	Type	Quantity	Frequency	Remarks

List of Nursing Diagnosis/Problems/Need Identified According to Priority

1. ____
2. ____
3. ____
4. ____
5. ____

Nursing Care Plan

ASSESSMENT Subjective Objective	Nursing diagnosis	GOALS Short-term Long-term	Implementation	Evaluation

Summary/Conclusion

Health Education

Reference

Date of submission:

Signature of subject In-charge

CASE PRESENTATION

■ HISTORY TAKING AND MENTAL STATUS EXAMINATION

Identification Data

Name	Age
Sex	Father/spouse
Education	Occupation
Income	Marital status
Religion	IP Number
Diagnosis	Address __________
	__________
	__________
	Informant:

Treatment received on arrival to hospital __________

____

____

History of Present Psychiatric Illness

What problem made you to come/bring to hospital?

____

When this symptoms started?

____

Any precipitating factors/aggravating factors?

____

Was the onset sudden or gradual?

____

How often does the problem occurs?

____

Has the problem occurs before?

____

Consider abnormal behavior, associated problem and disruptive behavior like suicide/homicide, changes in mood, thought, speech and abnormal perception __________

____

Reason for admission __________

Type of admission __________

Past Medical History

Any history of illness–hospitalization? If yes, history of diagnosis and treatment:

____

____

____

Any medical events, such as head injury, surgery, DM, hypertension, convulsion:

____

____

____

Past psychiatric illness (according to patient relatives):

____

____

____

____

____

____

____

____

____

____

____

History of hospitalization: Yes/No

Treatment taken: Yes/No

Psychological therapy:_______________________________________

Previous episode of any mental illness:

____

____

____

____

____

Family History of Psychiatric Illness

Sl. No.	Name of the family member	Age	Relationship with patient	Any psychiatric illness

Personal History

Perinatal history:

Antenatal period eventful/uneventful: _______________________

Exposure to radiation/drug/infection: _______________________

Natural birth, premature/normal/delivery/forceps delivery/caesarian section/instrumental delivery.

Birth cry: Immediate/delayed

Bonding: Immediate/delayed

Reaction of parents to childbirth: _______________________

Separation from mother: Yes/No

Postnatal complications:

Under–weight/infection/separations/underweight/infection/delayed breastfeeding: _______________________

Childhood history:

Parent relationship with the child: Harmonious/disturbed

Developmental milestone as per age: Normal/delayed

Relationship with family members: Normal/disturbed

Immunization received as per schedule: Yes/No

Feeding: Breastfeeding/artificial mode

Weaning: Response to weaning _______________________

Behavior: Temper tantrum/thumb sucking/stuttering/head banging/nail biting/night mares.

Educational history:

Academic achievement: Normal/underachiever

Extracurricular activity: Normal/underachiever

Relationship with teacher: Good/disturbed

Attendance to school: Adequate/frequent absent

Relationship with peers: Normal/not adjusting

Attitude towards schooling: Positive/Negative

Reason for discontinuing study if any: _______________________

Play history:

Participate in games sports: Yes/No. If yes, like to play individual/with group.

Relationship with playmates: Good/not adjustable

Puberty:

Age at menarche _______________________ Reaction to menarche _______________________

Regularity of cycle _______________________ Duration of flow _______________________

Occupational history:

Job started at what age: _______________________

Relationship with superior/colleagues/subordinate: Satisfactory/not satisfactory: _______________________

Sexual and marital history:

Type of marriage ____

Duration of marriage____

Relationship with spouse____

Marital disharmony, if any: _______________________________________

Interest and hobbies:

Relationship with neighbors: ______________________________________

Hobbies: ____

Premorbid personality:

Predominant mood: Anxious/pessimistic/optimistic/stable/fluctuating.

Personality: Shy/suspicious/irritable/self–centered/impulsive/unconfidence/obsessional.

◼ PHYSICAL EXAMINATION

Vital signs: Temperature _______________Pulse_______________Respiration_______________BP_______________

Any significant changes in CVS System: _______________________________

Any significant changes in respiratory system: __________________________

Any significant changes in GI system: ________________________________

Any significant changes in musculoskeletal system: ______________________

Any significant changes in reproductive system: ________________________

Any significant changes in integumentary system: _______________________

Any significant changes in respiratory system_________________________

Any other medical problems ______________________________________

◼ MENTAL STATUS EXAMINATION

General Appearance

- **Level of grooming:** Normal/stability dressing/overdressed/idiosyncratically dressed.
- **Level of cleanliness:** Adequate/inadequate/overtly clean
- **Level of consciousness:** Fully conscious/alert/drowsy/stupors/comatose
- **Mode of hospital admission:** Came to hospital willingly/persuaded/brought using physical force
- **Cooperativeness:** Normal/more than so/less than so
- **Eye to eye contact:** Normal/increased/decreased
- **Psychomotor activity:** Normal/increased/decreased
- **Rapport:** Spontaneous/difficult/not to establish
- **Gesture:** Grimace/tics/mannerism
- **Posturing:** Stereotype/tremors/extrapyramidal
- **Other movement:** Stereotype/tremors/extrapyramidal
- **Other catatonic phenomena:** Automatic obedience/negativism/excessive cooperation/waxy flexibility/echopraxia/echolalia.
- **Conversion and disassociate sign:** Yes/no
- **Compulsive act or rituals:** Yes/no
- **Hallucinatory behavior:** Yes/no

Speech

- **Initiation:** Spontaneous/speak when spoken/minimal/mute
- **Reaction time:** Normal/delayed/shortened/difficulty
- **Rate:** Normal/delayed
- **Tone:** Normal variation/monotonous
- **Others:** Rhyming/echolalia/neologism

Mood and Affect

- **Mood:** Angry/hopeless/retarded/thought block/flight of ideas
- **Affect:** Appropriate to mood/blunt/flat. If inappropriate, explain patient expression

____

____

Thinking and Perception

- **Stream of thought:**
    - Pressure of thought: Unusually rapid/abundant/varied.
    - Poverty of thoughts: Unusually slow/few or unvaried thoughts.
    - Blocking of thoughts: Abrupt/complete emptying of mind.
- **Form of thought:** Associative looseness/flight of ideas/incoherent/perseveration
- **Thought content:** Preoccupations/morbid thoughts/obsession/compulsion/delusion
  If delusion present mention the type: ____
- **Perceptual disturbances:**
    - Hallucinations/illusions. If present, mention the type _______________________________
    - Depersonalization/derealization

Orientation

- **Time:** Normal/impaired
- **Place:** Normal/impaired
- **Person:** Normal/impaired

Attention and Concentration

- **Attention:** Normal/Impaired
- **Concentration:** Normally sustained/sustained with difficulty

Memory

- **Immediate:** Intact/absent
- **Recent:** Intact/absent
- **Remote:** Intact/absent

Insight

- **Complete denial of illness:** Yes/No
- **Slight awareness of illness but in denial:** Yes/No
- **Awareness of illness but blaming others:** Yes/No
- **Intellectual insight:** Yes/No
- **True emotional insight:** Yes/No

Judgement

- **Personal judgment:** Intact/impaired
- **Social judgment:** Intact/impaired
- **Test judgment:** Intact/impaired

Book Picture and Patient Condition Comparison

Book picture	Patient condition
Etiology	
Psychopathology	
Clinical manifestation	
Investigation	
Diagnosis	
Psychopharmacology management	

Drug Study

Name of the drug	Dosage and frequency	Route	Action	Side effect	Nursing intervention

Diet Plan

24 hours Nutritional Requirements

Type of diet required (snacks, lunch, dinner)

Time	Type	Quantity	Frequency	Remarks

List of Nursing Diagnosis/Problems/Need Identified According to Priority

1. ____
2. ____
3. ____
4. ____
5. ____

Nursing Care Plan

ASSESSMENT Subjective Objective	Nursing diagnosis	GOALS Short-term Long-term	Implementation	Evaluation

Summary/Conclusion

Health Education

Reference

Date of submission: **Signature of subject In-charge**

DRUG STUDY

Name of the Patient: _________________________ **Diagnosis:** _________________________

Name of the drug	Route of administration	Dosage and frequency	Indication	Contraindication	Adverse reaction	Nursing intervention

Date of submission: **Signature of subject supervisor:**

PROCESS RECORDING: I

Identification Data

Name	Age
Sex	Father/spouse
Education	Occupation
Income	Marital status
Religion	IP Number
Diagnosis	Address __________
	__________
	__________
	__________
	Informant: __________

Treatment received on arrival to hospital __________
____
____
____

Date and time of process recording: __________

Patient problem: __________

Objective of process recording: __________

Preparation of patient: __________

Starting time of interaction: __________

Record of Interaction

Nurses interaction/verbatim	Patient response	Inference

Time completion of process recording: ____

Fixing the time and place for next interview: _______________________________________

Summary of inferences: ____

____

____

____

Significant inferences informed to the concerned _____________________________________

____

____

____

____

____

____

____

____

____

____

____

____

Date of submission: **Signature of Subject In-charge:**

PROCESS RECORDING: 2

Identification Data

Name	Age
Sex	Father/spouse
Education	Occupation
Income	Marital status
Religion	IP Number
Diagnosis	Address ______________________ ______________________ ______________________ ______________________ Informant: ______________

Treatment received on arrival to hospital ____
____
____
____

Date and time of process recording: ____

Patient problem: ____

Objective of process recording: ____

Preparation of patient: ____

Starting time of interaction: ____

Record of Interaction

Nurses interaction/verbatim	Patient response	Inference

Time completion of process recording: ____

Fixing the time and place for next interview: ____

Summary of inferences: ____

____

____

____

Significant inferences informed to the concerned ____

____

____

____

____

____

____

____

____

____

____

____

Date of submission: **Signature of Subject In-charge:**

MENTAL STATUS EXAMINATION: 1

■ IDENTIFICATION DATA

Name	Age
Sex	Father/spouse
Education	Occupation
Income	Marital status
Religion	IP Number
Diagnosis	Address ______________________ Informant: ______________________
Treatment received on arrival to hospital ______________________ 	

■ MENTAL STATUS EXAMINATION

General Appearance

- **Level of grooming:** Normal/stability dressing/overdressed/idiosyncratically dressed.
- **Level of cleanliness:** Adequate/inadequate/overtly clean
- **Level of consciousness:** Fully conscious/alert/drowsy/stupors/comatose
- **Mode of hospital admission:** Came to hospital willingly/persuaded/brought using physical force
- **Cooperativeness:** Normal/more than so/less than so
- **Eye to eye contact:** Normal/increased/decreased
- **Psychomotor activity:** Normal/increased/decreased
- **Rapport:** Spontaneous/difficult/not to establish
- **Gesture:** Grimace/tics/mannerism
- **Posturing:** Stereotype/tremors/extrapyramidal
- **Other movement:** Stereotype/tremors/extrapyramidal
- **Other catatonic phenomena:** Automatic obedience/negativism/excessive cooperation/waxy flexibility/echopraxia/echolalia.
- **Conversion and disassociate sign:** Yes/No
- **Compulsive act or rituals:** Yes/No
- **Hallucinatory behavior:** Yes/No

Speech

- **Initiation:** Spontaneous/speak when spoken/minimal/mute
- **Reaction time:** Normal/delayed/shortened/difficulty
- **Rate:** Normal/delayed
- **Tone:** Normal variation/monotonous
- **Others:** Rhyming/echolalia/neologism

Mood and Affect

- **Mood:** Angry/hopeless/retarded/thought block/flight of ideas
- **Affect:** Appropriate to mood/blunt/flat. If inappropriate, explain patient expression

---

Thinking and Perception

- **Stream of thought:**
  - Pressure of thought: Unusually rapid/abundant/varied.
  - Poverty of thoughts: Unusually slow/few or unvaried thoughts.
  - Blocking of thoughts: Abrupt/complete emptying of mind.
- **Form of thought:** Associative looseness/flight of ideas/incoherent/perseveration
- **Thought content:** Preoccupations/morbid thoughts/obsession/compulsion/delusion
  If delusion present mention the type: _______________________________________
- **Perceptual disturbances:**
  - Hallucinations/illusions. If present, mention the type _______________________________
  - Depersonalization/derealization

Orientation

- **Time:** Normal/impaired
- **Place:** Normal/impaired
- **Person:** Normal/impaired

Attention and Concentration

- **Attention:** Normal/impaired
- **Concentration:** Normally sustained/sustained with difficulty

Memory

- **Immediate:** Intact/absent
- **Recent:** Intact/absent
- **Remote:** Intact/absent

Insight

- **Complete denial of illness:** Yes/No
- **Slight awareness of illness but in denial:** Yes/No
- **Awareness of illness but blaming others:** Yes/No
- **Intellectual insight:** Yes/No
- **True emotional insight:** Yes/No

Judgment

- **Personal judgment:** Intact/impaired
- **Social judgment:** Intact/impaired
- **Test judgment:** Intact/impaired

Date of submission: **Signature of subject In-charge:**

MENTAL STATUS EXAMINATION: 2

■ IDENTIFICATION DATA

Name	Age
Sex	Father/spouse
Education	Occupation
Income	Marital status
Religion	IP Number
Diagnosis	Address ___________________ Informant: ___________________
Treatment received on arrival to hospital _______________________ 	

■ MENTAL STATUS EXAMINATION

General Appearance

- **Level of grooming:** Normal/stability dressing/overdressed/idiosyncratically dressed.
- **Level of cleanliness:** Adequate/inadequate/overtly clean
- **Level of consciousness:** Fully conscious/alert/drowsy/stupors/comatose
- **Mode of hospital admission:** Came to hospital willingly/persuaded/brought using physical force
- **Cooperativeness:** Normal/more than so/less than so
- **Eye to eye contact:** Normal/increased/decreased
- **Psychomotor activity:** Normal/increased/decreased
- **Rapport:** Spontaneous/difficult/not to establish
- **Gesture:** Grimace/tics/mannerism
- **Posturing:** Stereotype/tremors/extrapyramidal
- **Other movement:** Stereotype/tremors/extrapyramidal
- **Other catatonic phenomena:** Automatic obedience/negativism/excessive cooperation/waxy flexibility/echopraxia/echolalia.
- **Conversion and disassociate sign:** Yes/No
- **Compulsive act or rituals:** Yes/No
- **Hallucinatory behavior:** Yes/No

Speech

- **Initiation:** Spontaneous/speak when spoken/minimal/mute
- **Reaction time:** Normal/delayed/shortened/difficulty
- **Rate:** Normal/delayed
- **Tone:** Normal variation/monotonous
- **Others:** Rhyming/echolalia/neologism

Mood and Affect

- **Mood:** Angry/hopeless/retarded/thought block/flight of ideas
- **Affect:** Appropriate to mood/blunt/flat. If inappropriate, explain patient expression

Thinking and Perception

- **Stream of thought:**
    - Pressure of thought: Unusually rapid/abundant/varied.
    - Poverty of thoughts: Unusually slow/few or unvaried thoughts.
    - Blocking of thoughts: Abrupt/complete emptying of mind.
- **Form of thought:** Associative looseness/flight of ideas/incoherent/perseveration
- **Thought content:** Preoccupations/morbid thoughts/obsession/compulsion/delusion
  If delusion present mention the type: ____
- **Perceptual disturbances:**
    - Hallucinations/illusions. If present, mention the type _______________________________
    - Depersonalization/derealization

Orientation

- **Time:** Normal/impaired
- **Place:** Normal/impaired
- **Person:** Normal/impaired

Attention and Concentration

- **Attention:** Normal/impaired
- **Concentration:** Normally sustained/sustained with difficulty

Memory

- **Immediate:** Intact/absent
- **Recent:** Intact/absent
- **Remote:** Intact/absent

Insight

- **Complete denial of illness:** Yes/No
- **Slight awareness of illness but in denial:** Yes/No
- **Awareness of illness but blaming others:** Yes/No
- **Intellectual insight:** Yes/No
- **True emotional insight:** Yes/No

Judgment

- **Personal judgment:** Intact/impaired
- **Social judgment:** Intact/impaired
- **Test judgment:** Intact/impaired

Date of submission: **Signature of subject In-charge:**

MENTAL STATUS EXAMINATION: 3

■ IDENTIFICATION DATA

Name	Age
Sex	Father/spouse
Education	Occupation
Income	Marital status
Religion	IP Number
Diagnosis	Address ______________
	Informant: ______________
Treatment received on arrival to hospital ______________	

■ MENTAL STATUS EXAMINATION

General Appearance

- **Level of grooming:** Normal/stability dressing/overdressed/idiosyncratically dressed.
- **Level of cleanliness:** Adequate/inadequate/overtly clean
- **Level of consciousness:** Fully conscious/alert/drowsy/stupors/comatose
- **Mode of hospital admission:** Came to hospital willingly/persuaded/brought using physical force
- **Cooperativeness:** Normal/more than so/less than so
- **Eye to eye contact:** Normal/increased/decreased
- **Psychomotor activity:** Normal/increased/decreased
- **Rapport:** Spontaneous/difficult/not to establish
- **Gesture:** Grimace/tics/mannerism
- **Posturing:** Stereotype/tremors/extrapyramidal
- **Other movement:** Stereotype/tremors/extrapyramidal
- **Other catatonic phenomena:** Automatic obedience/negativism/excessive cooperation/waxy flexibility/echopraxia/echolalia.
- **Conversion and disassociate sign:** Yes/No
- **Compulsive act or rituals:** Yes/No
- **Hallucinatory behavior:** Yes/No

Speech

- **Initiation:** Spontaneous/speak when spoken/minimal/mute
- **Reaction time:** Normal/delayed/shortened/difficulty
- **Rate:** Normal/delayed
- **Tone:** Normal variation/monotonous
- **Others:** Rhyming/echolalia/neologism

Mood and Affect

- **Mood:** Angry/hopeless/retarded/thought block/flight of ideas
- **Affect:** Appropriate to mood/blunt/flat. If inappropriate, explain patient expression

Thinking and Perception

- **Stream of thought:**
    - Pressure of thought: Unusually rapid/abundant/varied.
    - Poverty of thoughts: Unusually slow/few or unvaried thoughts.
    - Blocking of thoughts: Abrupt/complete emptying of mind.
- **Form of thought:** Associative looseness/flight of ideas/incoherent/perseveration
- **Thought content:** Preoccupations/morbid thoughts/obsession/compulsion/delusion
  If delusion present mention the type: ____
- **Perceptual disturbances:**
    - Hallucinations/illusions. If present, mention the type _______________________________
    - Depersonalization/derealization

Orientation

- **Time:** Normal/impaired
- **Place:** Normal/impaired
- **Person:** Normal/impaired

Attention and Concentration

- **Attention:** Normal/impaired
- **Concentration:** Normally sustained/sustained with difficulty

Memory

- **Immediate:** Intact/absent
- **Recent:** Intact/absent
- **Remote:** Intact/absent

Insight

- **Complete denial of illness:** Yes/No
- **Slight awareness of illness but in denial:** Yes/No
- **Awareness of illness but blaming others:** Yes/No
- **Intellectual insight:** Yes/No
- **True emotional insight:** Yes/No

Judgment

- **Personal judgment:** Intact/impaired
- **Social judgment:** Intact/impaired
- **Test judgment:** Intact/impaired

Date of submission: **Signature of subject In-charge**

MENTAL STATUS EXAMINATION: 4

■ IDENTIFICATION DATA

Name	Age
Sex	Father/spouse
Education	Occupation
Income	Marital status
Religion	IP Number
Diagnosis	Address ___________________________ ___________________________ ___________________________ ___________________________ Informant: ___________________________ ___________________________
Treatment received on arrival to hospital ____ ____ ____ ____	

■ MENTAL STATUS EXAMINATION

General Appearance

- **Level of grooming:** Normal/stability dressing/overdressed/idiosyncratically dressed.
- **Level of cleanliness:** Adequate/inadequate/overtly clean
- **Level of consciousness:** Fully conscious/alert/drowsy/stupors/comatose
- **Mode of hospital admission:** Came to hospital willingly/persuaded/brought using physical force
- **Cooperativeness:** Normal/more than so/less than so
- **Eye to eye contact:** Normal/increased/decreased
- **Psychomotor activity:** Normal/increased/decreased
- **Rapport:** Spontaneous/difficult/not to establish
- **Gesture:** Grimace/tics/mannerism
- **Posturing:** Stereotype/tremors/extrapyramidal
- **Other movement:** Stereotype/tremors/extrapyramidal
- **Other catatonic phenomena:** Automatic obedience/negativism/excessive cooperation/waxy flexibility/echopraxia/echolalia.
- **Conversion and disassociate sign:** Yes/No
- **Compulsive act or rituals:** Yes/No
- **Hallucinatory behavior:** Yes/No

Speech

- **Initiation:** Spontaneous/speak when spoken/minimal/mute
- **Reaction time:** Normal/delayed/shortened/difficulty
- **Rate:** Normal/delayed
- **Tone:** Normal variation/monotonous
- **Others:** Rhyming/echolalia/neologism

Mood and Affect

- **Mood:** Angry/hopeless/retarded/thought block/flight of ideas
- **Affect:** Appropriate to mood/blunt/flat. If inappropriate, explain patient expression

Thinking and Perception

- **Stream of thought:**
    - Pressure of thought: Unusually rapid/abundant/varied.
    - Poverty of thoughts: Unusually slow/few or unvaried thoughts.
    - Blocking of thoughts: Abrupt/complete emptying of mind.
- **Form of thought:** Associative looseness/flight of ideas/incoherent/perseveration
- **Thought content:** Preoccupations/morbid thoughts/obsession/compulsion/delusion
  If delusion present mention the type: ____
- **Perceptual disturbances:**
    - Hallucinations/illusions. If present, mention the type _______________________________
    - Depersonalization/derealization

Orientation

- **Time:** Normal/impaired
- **Place:** Normal/impaired
- **Person:** Normal/impaired

Attention and Concentration

- **Attention:** Normal/impaired
- **Concentration:** Normally sustained/sustained with difficulty

Memory

- **Immediate:** Intact/absent
- **Recent:** Intact/absent
- **Remote:** Intact/absent

Insight

- **Complete denial of illness:** Yes/No
- **Slight awareness of illness but in denial:** Yes/No
- **Awareness of illness but blaming others:** Yes/No
- **Intellectual insight:** Yes/No
- **True emotional insight:** Yes/No

Judgment

- **Personal judgment:** Intact/impaired
- **Social judgment:** Intact/impaired
- **Test judgment:** Intact/impaired

Date of submission: **Signature of subject In-charge**

PEDIATRIC WARD

NURSING CARE PLAN: 1

■ IDENTIFICATION DATA

Name of the child:	IP No.:
Age:	Gender:
Mother name:	Father name:
Education:	Occupation of parents Father:____________Mother: ____________
Income:	
Religion:	Name of informant: Relationship with child:
Language spoken:	
Diagnosis:	Address: ______________________________ ______________________________ ______________________________ ______________________________
Treatment received on arrival to hospital ____	
Name of the treating Doctor:	

■ HISTORY OF PRESENT ILLNESS

Ask any or all of the following as appropriate and write a summary

Reason for visit:	Manner of onset: Gradual/sudden
Onset: ________________ Location: ________________ Duration: ________________ Aggravating factors: ________________ Relieving factors: ________________ Present complaints:	
How often the problem occurs?	Investigation done on time of admission:
Treatment given during admission:	Provisional diagnosis:

■ HISTORY OF PREVIOUS ILLNESS

Child birth history: ____

____

____

____

____

Significant History of Mother During Pregnancy

Length of pregnancy: ____

Maternal health medication taken: _____________________________________

Significant History of Mother During Delivery

Duration of labor: ____

Nature of delivery: ____

Birth weight: ____

Type of feeding: ____

Previous illness: ____

Immunization History

Immunization given: ____

Due to give: ____

Growth and Development

Weight: ____

Height: ____

Skin fold thickness: ____

Head circumference: ____

Chest circumference: ____

Mid–arm circumference: ____

Social, emotional and language development: ______________________________

____

____

Milestone development: ____

____

____

____

Gross motor development: ____

____

____

Fine motor development: ____

____

____

____

Immunization status: ____

____

____

____

Dietary pattern: _______________________________

Play habit: ___________________________________

Toilet training: _______________________________

Sleep pattern: ________________________________

Nutrition History

Dietary pattern: _______________________________

Appetite change: ______________________________

Weight change: _______________________________

Nausea: ______________________________________

Vomiting: ____________________________________

Dysphasia: ___________________________________

Condition of dentures upper/lower: _________________________

Normal eating pattern (likes and dislikes): ____________________

Family History

Sl. No.	Name of the family member	Age	Sex	Significant disease, e.g., DM, TB, Epilepsy, etc.

Family Tree

■ PHYSICAL EXAMINATION

Approach and preparation: Observing readiness to cooperate, smiling, talking, making eye contact and allowing nurse (student) to touch him or her are all positive clues to readiness.

General appearance:

- Note whether child appear well, ill, in acute/distress or chronically ill:

  ____

- Facial expression and appearance:

  ____

- Observe posture, position and body movement (body language gives important clues to emotional state):

  ____

- Observe behavior and activity: Child is alert/lethargic/withdrawn/dull
- Note movement of child passively moving _____________________ any abnormality _____________________
- **Vital signs:** Pulse _____________________ Temperature _____________________
  Respiration _____________________ Blood pressure _____________________
- Observe personal hygiene and grooming (Note state of cleanliness):
  - Note any unusual body odors _____________________
  - Condition of hair _____________________
  - Condition of nail _____________________
  - Condition of teeth _____________________
  - Condition of clothing _____________________
- Any changes in skin color _____________________
- Pigmentation/pallor/jaundice/cyanosis/lymph nodes.
- Head:
  - Measure head circumference _____________________
  - Observe obvious swelling _____________________

- **Bulging fontanels:** _______________________________
- **Neck:**
    - Inspect neck for size and symmetry________________________________
    - Excessively small lower jaw/large lower jaw.
- Palpate trachea note any abnormalities________________________________
- **Eyes:** Inspect eyes for position, spacing, alignment and symmetry__________________pupil size ______________________shape______________and movement____________
- **Ears:** Inspect pinna ______________any discharge ____________pain __________
- **Nose:** size____________shape____________any abnormalities __________
- Teeth________________________
- Mouth and throat ________________
- **Observe:** Lips color____________texture____________excessive salivation__________
- Observe mucous membrane, gums, tongue any abnormalities__________
- Inspect breast, nipple and areola for shape, size, and color. Note any abnormality.

 ____

- Observe any coughing, wheezing, hoarseness: ________________

Respiratory System

- **Rate:** ________________ **Characteristics:** ________________
- **Cough:** Dyspnea/wheezing/coughs blood (hemoptysis)
- **Cyanosis:** Pain on breathing.

    COMMENTS ____

 ____

- **Palpate chest:**________________________________
- **Assess expansion of chest:** ________________________
- **Auscultate breath sounds and note:** ____________________

Cardiac System

- **Heart:** Palpate anterior chest wall and note________________

Abdomen

- **Abdomen:** Auscultate bowel sounds________________
- **Palpate abdomen organs:** Note any tenderness or mass ____________
- **Genitalia:** Observe size of penis, inspect for swelling, skin lesion or inflammation of glans and shaft

 ____

Investigation Done

Date	Name of the investigation	Normal values	Patients values/result	Significance

Diagnosis (Final) ________________________________

Drug Management

Sl. No.	Name of the drug	Dosage and frequency	Route	Action	Side effect	Nursing intervention

Diet Plan

24 hours Nutritional Requirements

____

____

____

____

____

____

Nursing Care Plan

ASSESSMENT Subjective Objective	Nursing diagnosis	GOALS Short-term Long-term	Implementation	Evaluation

Summary/Conclusion

Health Education

Reference

Date of submission: **Signature of subject In-charge**

NURSING CARE PLAN: 2

■ IDENTIFICATION DATA

Name of the child:	IP No.:
Age:	Gender:
Mother name:	Father name:
Education:	Occupation of parents Father:______________Mother:______________
Income:	
Religion:	Name of informant: Relationship with child:
Language spoken:	
Diagnosis:	Address: __________________________ __________________________ __________________________ __________________________
Treatment received on arrival to hospital ______________________________ ____ ____ ____	
Name of the treating Doctor:	

■ HISTORY OF PRESENT ILLNESS

Ask any or all of the following as appropriate and write a summary

Reason for visit:	Manner of onset: Gradual/sudden
Onset: __________ Location: __________ Duration: __________ Aggravating factors: __________ Relieving factors: __________ Present complaints:	
How often the problem occurs?	Investigation done on time of admission:
Treatment given during admission:	Provisional diagnosis:

■ HISTORY OF PREVIOUS ILLNESS

Child birth history: _______________________

____

____

____

Significant History of Mother During Pregnancy

Length of pregnancy: _______________________

Maternal health medication taken: _______________________

Significant History of Mother During Delivery

Duration of labor: _______________________

Nature of delivery: _______________________

Birth weight: _______________________

Type of feeding: _______________________

Previous illness: _______________________

Immunization History

Immunization given: _______________________

Due to give: _______________________

Growth and Development

Weight: _______________________

Height: _______________________

Skin fold thickness: _______________________

Head circumference: _______________________

Chest circumference: _______________________

Mid–arm circumference: _______________________

Social, emotional and language development: _______________________

____

____

Milestone development: _______________________

____

____

____

Gross motor development: _______________________

____

____

Fine motor development: ____

____

____

____

Immunization status: ____

____

____

____

Dietary pattern: ___________________________________

Play habit: _______________________________________

Toilet training: ___________________________________

Sleep pattern: ____________________________________

Nutrition History

Dietary pattern: ___________________________________

Appetite change: __________________________________

Weight change: ___________________________________

Nausea: ____

Vomiting: ____

Dysphasia: _______________________________________

Condition of dentures upper/lower: _________________

Normal eating pattern (likes and dislikes): _____________

Family History

Sl. No.	Name of the family member	Age	Sex	Significant disease, e.g., DM, TB, Epilepsy, etc.

Family Tree

■ PHYSICAL EXAMINATION

Approach and preparation: Observing readiness to cooperate, smiling, talking, making eye contact and allowing nurse (student) to touch him or her are all positive clues to readiness.

General appearance:
- Note whether child appear well, ill, in acute/distress or chronically ill:

  ____

- Facial expression and appearance:

  ____

- Observe posture, position and body movement (body language gives important clues to emotional state):

  ____

- Observe behavior and activity: Child is alert/lethargic/withdrawn/dull
- Note movement of child passively moving _______________ any abnormality _______________
- **Vital signs:** Pulse _______________ Temperature _______________

  Respiration _______________ Blood pressure _______________
- Observe personal hygiene and grooming (Note state of cleanliness):
    - Note any unusual body odors _______________
    - Condition of hair _______________
    - Condition of nail _______________
    - Condition of teeth _______________
    - Condition of clothing _______________
- Any changes in skin color _______________
- Pigmentation/pallor/jaundice/cyanosis/lymph nodes.
- Head:
    - Measure head circumference _______________
    - Observe obvious swelling _______________

- **Bulging fontanels:** _______________________
- **Neck:**
  - Inspect neck for size and symmetry_______________________
  - Excessively small lower jaw/large lower jaw.
- Palpate trachea note any abnormalities_______________________
- **Eyes:** Inspect eyes for position, spacing, alignment and symmetry_______________________pupil size _______________________shape_______________________and movement_______________________
- **Ears:** Inspect pinna _______________________any discharge _______________________pain _______________________
- **Nose:** size_______________________shape_______________________any abnormalities _______________________
- Teeth_______________________
- Mouth and throat _______________________
- **Observe:** Lips color_______________________texture_______________________excessive salivation_______________________
- Observe mucous membrane, gums, tongue any abnormalities_______________________
- Inspect breast, nipple and areola for shape, size, and color. Note any abnormality.
  ____
- Observe any coughing, wheezing, hoarseness: _______________________

Respiratory System

- **Rate:** _______________________ **Characteristics:** _______________________
- **Cough:** Dyspnea/wheezing/coughs blood (hemoptysis)
- **Cyanosis:** Pain on breathing.

  COMMENTS _______________________
  ____

- **Palpate chest:**_______________________
- **Assess expansion of chest:** _______________________
- **Auscultate breath sounds and note:** _______________________

Cardiac System

- **Heart:** Palpate anterior chest wall and note_______________________

Abdomen

- **Abdomen:** Auscultate bowel sounds_______________________
- **Palpate abdomen organs:** Note any tenderness or mass _______________________
- **Genitalia:** Observe size of penis, inspect for swelling, skin lesion or inflammation of glans and shaft
  ____

Investigation Done

Date	Name of the investigation	Normal values	Patients values/result	Significance

Diagnosis (Final) _______________________

Drug Management

Sl. No.	Name of the drug	Dosage and frequency	Route	Action	Side effect	Nursing intervention

Diet Plan

24 hours Nutritional Requirements

Nursing Care Plan

ASSESSMENT Subjective Objective	Nursing diagnosis	GOALS Short-term Long-term	Implementation	Evaluation

Summary/Conclusion

Health Education

Reference

Date of submission: **Signature of subject In-charge**

CASE STUDY

■ IDENTIFICATION DATA

Name of the child:	IP No.:
Age:	Gender:
Mother name:	Father name:
Education:	Occupation of parents Father:_______________Mother:___________
Income:	
Religion:	Name of informant: Relationship with child:
Language spoken:	
Diagnosis:	Address: _______________________ _______________________ _______________________ _______________________
Treatment received on arrival to hospital ________________________ ____ ____ ____	
Name of the treating Doctor:	

■ HISTORY OF PRESENT ILLNESS

Ask any or all of the following as appropriate and write a summary

Reason for visit:.	Manner of onset: Gradual/sudden
Onset: ___________ Location: _____________ Duration: __________ Aggravating factors: ______________Relieving factors: __________ Present complaints:	
How often the problem occurs?	Investigation done on time of admission:
Treatment given during admission:	Provisional diagnosis:

■ HISTORY OF PREVIOUS ILLNESS

Child birth history: _______________________________

____

____

____

Significant History of Mother During Pregnancy

Length of pregnancy: _______________________________

Maternal health medication taken: _______________________________

Significant History of Mother During Delivery

Duration of labor: _______________________________

Nature of delivery: _______________________________

Birth weight: _______________________________

Type of feeding: _______________________________

Previous illness: _______________________________

Immunization History

Immunization given: _______________________________

Due to give: _______________________________

Growth and Development

Weight: _______________________________

Height: _______________________________

Skin fold thickness: _______________________________

Head circumference: _______________________________

Chest circumference: _______________________________

Mid–arm circumference: _______________________________

Social, emotional and language development: _______________________________

____

____

Milestone development: _______________________________

____

____

____

Gross motor development: _______________________________

____

____

Fine motor development: ____

____

____

____

Immunization status: ____

____

____

____

Dietary pattern: _______________________________

Play habit: ____________________________________

Toilet training: _______________________________

Sleep pattern: _________________________________

Nutrition History

Dietary pattern: _______________________________

Appetite change: ______________________________

Weight change: ________________________________

Nausea: _______________________________________

Vomiting: _____________________________________

Dysphasia: ____________________________________

Condition of dentures upper/lower: ___________________

Normal eating pattern (likes and dislikes): _____________

Family History

Sl. No.	Name of the family member	Age	Sex	Significant disease, e.g., DM, TB, Epilepsy, etc.

Family Tree

■ PHYSICAL EXAMINATION

Approach and preparation: Observing readiness to cooperate, smiling, talking, making eye contact and allowing nurse (student) to touch him or her are all positive clues to readiness.

General appearance:

- Note whether child appear well, ill, in acute/distress or chronically ill:

  ____

- Facial expression and appearance:

  ____

- Observe posture, position and body movement (body language gives important clues to emotional state):

  ____

- Observe behavior and activity: Child is alert/lethargic/withdrawn/dull
- Note movement of child passively moving _______________any abnormality_______________
- **Vital signs:** Pulse_______________Temperature _______________
  Respiration_______________Blood pressure_______________
- Observe personal hygiene and grooming (Note state of cleanliness):
  - Note any unusual body odors _______________
  - Condition of hair_______________
  - Condition of nail_______________
  - Condition of teeth_______________
  - Condition of clothing_______________
- Any changes in skin color_______________
- Pigmentation/pallor/jaundice/cyanosis/lymph nodes.
- Head:
  - Measure head circumference _______________
  - Observe obvious swelling_______________

- **Bulging fontanels:** _______________________________________
- **Neck:**
  - Inspect neck for size and symmetry____
  - Excessively small lower jaw/large lower jaw.
- Palpate trachea note any abnormalities____
- **Eyes:** Inspect eyes for position, spacing, alignment and symmetry________________________pupil size
  ________________________shape________________________and movement________________________
- **Ears:** Inspect pinna ________________any discharge ________________pain ________________
- **Nose:** size________________shape________________any abnormalities________________
- Teeth____
- Mouth and throat ________________________________
- **Observe:** Lips color________________texture________________excessive salivation________________
- Observe mucous membrane, gums, tongue any abnormalities____
- Inspect breast, nipple and areola for shape, size, and color. Note any abnormality.

  ____

- Observe any coughing, wheezing, hoarseness: ________________________________

Respiratory System

- **Rate:** ________________________ **Characteristics:** ________________________
- **Cough:** Dyspnea/wheezing/coughs blood (hemoptysis)
- **Cyanosis:** Pain on breathing.

  COMMENTS ____

  ____

- **Palpate chest:** ____
- **Assess expansion of chest:** ____
- **Auscultate breath sounds and note:** ____

Cardiac System

- **Heart:** Palpate anterior chest wall and note____

Abdomen

- **Abdomen:** Auscultate bowel sounds____
- **Palpate abdomen organs:** Note any tenderness or mass ________________________________
- **Genitalia:** Observe size of penis, inspect for swelling, skin lesion or inflammation of glans and shaft

  ____

Comparing Theory Knowledge with Present Patient Condition

Knowledge of disease	As per theory knowledge	Present in patient
Definition		
Review related anatomy and physiology		

Knowledge of disease	As per theory knowledge	Present in patient
Etiology		
Diagnosis		
Clinical manifestation		
Diagnosis evaluation/ investigation		
Medical management		
Surgical management		
Dietary management		

Nursing Care Plan

ASSESSMENT Subjective Objective	Nursing diagnosis	GOALS Short-term Long-term	Implementation	Evaluation

Summary/Conclusion

Health Education

Reference

Date of submission: Signature of subject In-charge

CASE PRESENTATION

◼ IDENTIFICATION DATA

Name of the child:	IP No.:
Age:	Gender:
Mother name:	Father name:
Education:	Occupation of parents Father:________________Mother:_______________
Income:	
Religion:	Name of informant: Relationship with child:
Language spoken:	
Diagnosis:	Address: ________________________ ________________________ ________________________ ________________________
Treatment received on arrival to hospital ____________________________ ____ ____ ____	
Name of the treating Doctor:	

◼ HISTORY OF PRESENT ILLNESS

Ask any or all of the following as appropriate and write a summary

Reason for visit:	Manner of onset: Gradual/sudden
Onset: ___________Location: ___________Duration: ___________ Aggravating factors: ___________Relieving factors: ___________ Present complaints:	
How often the problem occurs?	Investigation done on time of admission:
Treatment given during admission:	Provisional diagnosis:

■ HISTORY OF PREVIOUS ILLNESS

Child birth history: ____

____

____

____

Significant History of Mother During Pregnancy

Length of pregnancy: ____

Maternal health medication taken: ______________________________________

Significant History of Mother During Delivery

Duration of labor: ____

Nature of delivery: ____

Birth weight: ____

Type of feeding: ____

Previous illness: ____

Immunization History

Immunization given: ____

Due to give: ____

Growth and Development

Weight: ____

Height: ____

Skin fold thickness: ____

Head circumference: ____

Chest circumference: ____

Mid–arm circumference: ____

Social, emotional and language development: ________________________________

____

____

Milestone development: ____

____

____

____

Gross motor development: ____

____

____

____

Fine motor development: ____

____

____

Immunization status: ____

____

____

____

Dietary pattern: _______________________________________

Play habit: ____

Toilet training: _______________________________________

Sleep pattern: ____

Nutrition History

Dietary pattern: _______________________________________

Appetite change: ______________________________________

Weight change: _______________________________________

Nausea: ____

Vomiting: ____

Dysphasia: ____

Condition of dentures upper/lower: ________________________

Normal eating pattern (likes and dislikes): ___________________

Family History

Sl. No.	Name of the family member	Age	Sex	Significant disease, e.g., DM, TB, Epilepsy, etc.

Family Tree

◼ PHYSICAL EXAMINATION

Approach and preparation: Observing readiness to cooperate, smiling, talking, making eye contact and allowing nurse (student) to touch him or her are all positive clues to readiness.

General appearance:

- Note whether child appear well, ill, in acute/distress or chronically ill:

  ____

- Facial expression and appearance:

  ____

- Observe posture, position and body movement (body language gives important clues to emotional state):

  ____

- Observe behavior and activity: Child is alert/lethargic/withdrawn/dull
- Note movement of child passively moving _______________________any abnormality_______________________
- **Vital signs:** Pulse_______________________Temperature_______________________

  Respiration_______________________Blood pressure_______________________
- Observe personal hygiene and grooming (Note state of cleanliness):
    - Note any unusual body odors _______________________
    - Condition of hair_______________________
    - Condition of nail_______________________
    - Condition of teeth_______________________
    - Condition of clothing_______________________
- Any changes in skin color_______________________
- Pigmentation/pallor/jaundice/cyanosis/lymph nodes.
- Head:
    - Measure head circumference _______________________
    - Observe obvious swelling_______________________

- **Bulging fontanels:** _______________________________
- **Neck:**
    - Inspect neck for size and symmetry____________________________________
    - Excessively small lower jaw/large lower jaw.
- Palpate trachea note any abnormalities____________________________________
- **Eyes:** Inspect eyes for position, spacing, alignment and symmetry________________________pupil size
  ____________________shape________________________and movement________________________
- **Ears:** Inspect pinna ________________any discharge ________________pain ________________
- **Nose:** size________________shape________________any abnormalities________________
- Teeth____
- Mouth and throat ________________________________
- **Observe:** Lips color________________texture________________excessive salivation________________
- Observe mucous membrane, gums, tongue any abnormalities________________________
- Inspect breast, nipple and areola for shape, size, and color. Note any abnormality.

  ____
- Observe any coughing, wheezing, hoarseness: ________________________________

Respiratory System

- **Rate:** ________________________ **Characteristics**: ________________________
- **Cough:** Dyspnea/wheezing/coughs blood (hemoptysis)
- **Cyanosis:** Pain on breathing.

  COMMENTS ____

  ____

- **Palpate chest:** ____
- **Assess expansion of chest:** ________________________________
- **Auscultate breath sounds and note:** ________________________________

Cardiac System

- **Heart:** Palpate anterior chest wall and note________________________________

Abdomen

- **Abdomen:** Auscultate bowel sounds________________________________
- **Palpate abdomen organs:** Note any tenderness or mass ________________________
- **Genitalia:** Observe size of penis, inspect for swelling, skin lesion or inflammation of glans and shaft

  ____

Comparing Theory Knowledge with Present Patient Condition

Knowledge of disease	As per theory knowledge	Present in patient
Definition		
Review related anatomy and physiology		

Knowledge of disease	As per theory knowledge	Present in patient
Etiology		
Diagnosis		
Clinical manifestation		
Diagnosis evaluation/ investigation		
Medical management		
Surgical management		
Dietary management		

Nursing Care Plan

ASSESSMENT Subjective Objective	Nursing diagnosis	GOALS Short-term Long-term	Implementation	Evaluation

Summary/Conclusion

Health Education

Reference

Date of submission: **Signature of subject In-charge**

DRUG STUDY

Name of the Patient: _______________________ Diagnosis: _______________________

Name of the drug	Route of administration	Dosage and frequency	Indication	Contraindication	Adverse reaction	Nursing intervention

Date of submission: **Signature of subject supervisor:**

OBSERVATION REPORT (NEWBORN): 1

Birth age: _____________________________ Date of birth: _____________________

Time of birth: _________________________ Weight: __________________________

Date of observation: _________________

Parameter	Signs and symptoms	Interval of observation			
Respiratory	Temperature				
	Heart rate				
	Weight				
	Sneezing				
General nervous system	Cry high-pitched				
	Cry inconsolable				
	Tremors				
	Abnormal muscle tone				
	Disorganized sucking				
	Feeding duration				
Gastrointestinal	Vomiting				
	Loose watery				
	Excoriation				

Summary

____

____

____

____

____

____

____

____

____

Date of submission: **Signature of subject In-charge:**

OBSERVATION REPORT (NEWBORN): 2

Birth age: _______________________________   Date of birth: _______________________________

Time of birth: _____________________________   Weight: _______________________________

Date of observation: _______________________

Parameter	Signs and symptoms	Interval of observation			
Respiratory	Temperature				
	Heart rate				
	Weight				
	Sneezing				
General nervous system	Cry high-pitched				
	Cry inconsolable				
	Tremors				
	Abnormal muscle tone				
	Disorganized sucking				
	Feeding duration				
Gastrointestinal	Vomiting				
	Loose watery				
	Excoriation				

Summary

____

____

____

____

____

____

____

____

____

Date of submission: **Signature of subject In-charge:**

GNM THIRD YEAR

Maternity Ward Requirement

■ THIRD YEAR

Sl. No.	Practical record	Requirement
	Maternity Ward	
1.	Nursing care plan	2+1
2.	Case study	1+1
3.	Case presentation	1+1
4.	Drug study	1+1
	Daily Diary: Rural and Urban Community	
1.	Health talk	2 each
2.	Family health talk nursing care plan	2 each
3.	Group project	1 each

MATERNITY WARD

NURSING CARE PLAN: 1

Name of the patient: _______________________________   IP number: _______________________________

Name of the hospital: _______________________________   Date of admission: _______________________________

Treating Doctor: _______________________________

Demographic Data

Name of the patient:	Age:
Name of husband:	Husband age:
Date of first visit:	Language spoken:
Education:	Occupation
Husband education:	Husband occupation:
Family income:	Address with contact number:

Present Pregnancy Complaints

Possible problems in all trimesters of pregnancy:
Headache/dizziness/visual disturbance/syncope/fatigue/nausea/vomiting/heart burn/shortness of breath/abdominal pain/vaginal bleeding/vaginal discharge/constipation/hemorrhoids/ankle edema

Bowel habits: Regular/irregular	**Skin:** Abdominal wall/groin/vulva/anal region
Lymphatic system: Enlarged gland/neck/axilla/groin/lymphangitis	**Vaginal discharge:** Red/white

Menstrual history:
Age at menarche: _______________________________
Regular/irregular: _______________________________
Duration: 3 days/5 days/8 days _______________________________

Past obstetric history:
Anemia/neonatal death/neonatal anomaly/gestational diabetes/hyperemesis gravidarum/incompetent cervix/polyhydramnios/postpartum depression/pregnancy-induced hypertension/preterm labor.

History of Present Pregnancy

Gestation at first week:	EDD:
LMP:	PARA/GRAVIDA:

G_______________________________ A_______________________________ P_______________________________ L_______________________________

Family History

Type of family: Nuclear/joint family

Family Composition

Sl. No.	Name	Relationship to the patient	Age	Sex	Education	Occupation	Health status

Family Tree:

Family History of Illness

Is there any family history of: Asthma/cancer/diabetes/epilepsy/hypertension/heart disease/hepatitis/hemophilia/ stroke/tuberculosis/mental disorders/thyroid or autoimmune disorders/aged grandparent and siblings alive? If yes, what is their current state of health? If no, state the cause of death and age of death ___________________________

____

____

____

Past History

History of Past Pregnancy

Sl. No.	Year and month	Pregnancy events	Labor events	Mode of delivery	Puerperium	Baby status

Past Health History

Abortion history: Pregnancy loss __________________________ Month and year__________________________ **Sex of the birth:** Male/female **Type of abortion:** Spontaneous/induced/term/preterm/ congenital abnormalities__________________	**Previous type of delivery:** Normal/vaginal/ forceps/cesarean section

Gynecological history: Abnormal PAP, any gynecological surgery/infertility.

Past Medical history:

Hypertension/DM/heart disease/rheumatic fever/mitral valve prolapse/thrombophlebitis/asthma/allergy/thyroid disorders/gonorrhea/herpes simplex/syphilis/heart disease/rheumatic fever.

Psychological history: Abuse/neglect.

Physical examination:

- Condition of ear__________nose__________teeth__________gums__________tonsils__________
- **Breast and nipple changes:** Tenderness/painful/warmth/presence of cyst. Nipple retraction/inverted/cracked.
- Heart sounds__________________________
- Lungs__________________________
- Spleen__________________________
- Liver__________________________
- **Skin changes:** Chloasma/linea nigra/striae (pink white). __________
- Anal changes (hemorrhoids, edema and type) __________

Antenatal examination:

General appearance:

Body built __________________________

Height__________________weight __________________

Vital signs: Temp__________Pulse__________Resp__________BP__________

Skin turgor: Moisture/dry

Face puffiness: Yes/No

Lips: Cyanosis/dryness

Ears: Discharge__________pain __________

Nose: Normal/septal defect/broad/flat nose.

Abdominal examination:
- **Inspection:** Uterine size___________shape___________fetal movement___________skin changes___________
- **Palpation:** Girth of the abdomen___________fundal height___________fundal palpation___________
  1st pelvic grip___________2nd pelvic grip___________3rd pelvic grip___________4th pelvic grip___________
- Auscultation FHR___________Right side___________Rate per minute/rhythm___________
  location___________position___________left side___________rate per minute.
  Rhythm___________location___________position___________

PV examination:

Cervix___________internal OS___________external OS___________dilation___________effacement
___________position___________presentation___________presenting part___________adequacy of
pelvis___________discharge___________

Other examination:
- **Blood group**___________Rh type___________Hb%___________BT___________CT___________
  VDRL___________HBs AG___________
- **Urine:** Sugar___________albumin___________micro___________

Present obstetrical history:

Type of delivery___________time of onset of labor pain ___________duration of labor ___________
medication given___________problem after delivery___________

Newborn examination:
- Alive/still birth
- Weight of the baby___________
- Sex of the baby___________
- **Activity:** Active/dull
- **Head to toe examination:**
  - *Head:* Distribution of hair___________ condition of hair ___________ condition of scalp ___________
  - *Face*___________presence of edema___________
  - *Ears:* Hearing capacity___________
  - *Eyes* any discharge/swelling/redness. Color of conjunctiva: Pink/pale
  - *Nose:* Any discharge/polyps
  - *Lips:* Moist or any cracks
  - *Tongue*___________
  - *Neck*___________Neck rigidity___________
  - *Chest and thorax:* Symmetry of movement___________breath sounds___________
  - *Extremities:* Range of motion___________

Apgar Scoring

Sl. No.	Sign	0	1–5 min	1	1–5 min	2	1–5 min
1.	Respiratory effort	Absent		Slow irregular, weak cry		Strong cry	
2.	Heart rate	Absent		Slow, less than 100		Over 100	
3.	Muscle tone	Limp		Some flexion of limb		Active movement	

Sl. No.	Sign	0	1–5 min	1	1–5 min	2	1–5 min
4.	Reflex response to flicking of foot	Absent		Facial grimace		Cry	
5.	Color	Blue pale		Body pink Limbs blue		Completely pink	

Score_____________

0–2: Severe asphyxia

3–4: Moderate asphyxia

5–7: No asphyxia

- Still born/macerated _________________________causes_________________________
  treatment at birth_________________________
- Birth injuries_________________________
- Congenital abnormalities_________________________
- Medication given_________________________

Investigation Done

Date	Name of the investigation	Normal values	Patients values/result	Significance

Diagnosis (Final) _________________________

Drug Management

Name of the drug	Dosage and frequency	Route	Indication	Action	Contraindication	Side effect	Nursing intervention

Diet Plan

24 hours Nutritional Requirements

____

____

____

____

Nursing Care Plan

ASSESSMENT Subjective Objective	Nursing diagnosis	GOALS Short-term Long-term	Implementation	Evaluation

Summary/Conclusion

Health Education

Reference

Date of submission: **Signature of subject In-charge:**

NURSING CARE PLAN: 2

Name of the patient: _________________________________ IP number: _______________________

Name of the hospital: _______________________________ Date of admission: _________________

Treating Doctor: ____________________

Demographic Data

Name of the patient:	Age:
Name of husband:	Husband age:
Date of first visit:	Language spoken:
Education:	Occupation
Husband education:	Husband occupation:
Family income:	Address with contact number:

Present Pregnancy Complaints

Possible problems in all trimesters of pregnancy:

Headache/dizziness/visual disturbance/syncope/fatigue/nausea/vomiting/heart burn/shortness of breath/abdominal pain/vaginal bleeding/vaginal discharge/constipation/hemorrhoids/ankle edema

Bowel habits: Regular/irregular	**Skin:** Abdominal wall/groin/vulva/anal region
Lymphatic system: Enlarged gland/neck/axilla/groin/lymphangitis	**Vaginal discharge:** Red/white

Menstrual history:

Age at menarche: _______________________________

Regular/irregular: ______________________________

Duration: 3 days/5 days/8 days ______________________

Past obstetric history:

Anemia/neonatal death/neonatal anomaly/gestational diabetes/hyperemesis gravidarum/incompetent cervix/polyhydramnios/postpartum depression/pregnancy-induced hypertension/preterm labor.

History of Present Pregnancy

Gestation at first week:	EDD:
LMP:	PARA/GRAVIDA:

G_________________________ A _________________________ P _________________________ L _________________________

Family History

Type of family: Nuclear/joint family

Family Composition

Sl. No.	Name	Relationship to the patient	Age	Sex	Education	Occupation	Health status

Family Tree:

Family History of Illness

Is there any family history of: Asthma/cancer/diabetes/epilepsy/hypertension/heart disease/hepatitis/hemophilia/ stroke/tuberculosis/mental disorders/thyroid or autoimmune disorders/aged grandparent and siblings alive? If yes, what is their current state of health? If no, state the cause of death and age of death ________________________

____

____

____

Past History

History of Past Pregnancy

Sl. No.	Year and month	Pregnancy events	Labor events	Mode of delivery	Puerperium	Baby status

Past Health History

Abortion history:	**Previous type of delivery:** Normal/vaginal/ forceps/cesarean section
Pregnancy loss _________________________ Month and year_________________________ **Sex of the birth:** Male/female **Type of abortion:** Spontaneous/induced/term/preterm/ congenital abnormalities_________________	

Gynecological history: Abnormal PAP, any gynecological surgery/infertility.

Past Medical history:

Hypertension/DM/heart disease/rheumatic fever/mitral valve prolapse/thrombophlebitis/asthma/allergy/thyroid disorders/gonorrhea/herpes simplex/syphilis/heart disease/rheumatic fever.

Psychological history: Abuse/neglect.

Physical examination:

- Condition of ear__________nose__________teeth__________gums__________tonsils__________
- **Breast and nipple changes:** Tenderness/painful/warmth/presence of cyst. Nipple retraction/inverted/cracked.
- Heart sounds_________________________
- Lungs_________________________
- Spleen_________________________
- Liver_________________________
- **Skin changes:** Chloasma/linea nigra/striae (pink white). _________________________
- Anal changes (hemorrhoids, edema and type) _________________________

Antenatal examination:

General appearance:

Body built _________________________

Height_________________________weight _________________________

Vital signs: Temp__________Pulse__________Resp__________BP__________

Skin turgor: Moisture/dry

Face puffiness: Yes/No

Lips: Cyanosis/dryness

Ears: Discharge_________________________pain _________________________

Nose: Normal/septal defect/broad/flat nose.

Abdominal examination:

- **Inspection:** Uterine size___________ shape___________ fetal movement___________ skin changes___________
- **Palpation:** Girth of the abdomen___________ fundal height___________ fundal palpation___________
  1st pelvic grip___________ 2nd pelvic grip___________ 3rd pelvic grip___________ 4th pelvic grip___________
- Auscultation FHR___________ Right side ___________ Rate per minute/rhythm___________
  location___________ position___________ left side___________ rate per minute.
  Rhythm___________ location___________ position___________

PV examination:

Cervix___________ internal OS___________ external OS___________ dilation___________ effacement
___________ position___________ presentation___________ presenting part___________ adequacy of
pelvis___________ discharge___________

Other examination:

- **Blood group**___________ Rh type___________ Hb%___________ BT___________ CT___________
  VDRL___________ HBs AG___________
- **Urine:** Sugar___________ albumin___________ micro___________

Present obstetrical history:

Type of delivery___________ time of onset of labor pain ___________ duration of labor ___________
medication given___________ problem after delivery___________

Newborn examination:

- Alive/still birth
- Weight of the baby___________
- Sex of the baby___________
- **Activity:** Active/dull
- **Head to toe examination:**
  - *Head:* Distribution of hair___________ condition of hair ___________ condition of scalp ___________
  - *Face*___________ presence of edema___________
  - *Ears:* Hearing capacity___________
  - *Eyes* any discharge/swelling/redness. Color of conjunctiva: Pink/pale
  - *Nose:* Any discharge/polyps
  - *Lips:* Moist or any cracks
  - *Tongue*___________
  - *Neck*___________ Neck rigidity___________
  - *Chest and thorax:* Symmetry of movement___________ breath sounds___________
  - *Extremities:* Range of motion___________

Apgar Scoring

Sl. No.	Sign	0	1–5 min	1	1–5 min	2	1–5 min
1.	Respiratory effort	Absent		Slow irregular, weak cry		Strong cry	
2.	Heart rate	Absent		Slow, less than 100		Over 100	
3.	Muscle tone	Limp		Some flexion of limb		Active movement	

Sl. No.	Sign	0	1–5 min	1	1–5 min	2	1–5 min
4.	Reflex response to flicking of foot	Absent		Facial grimace		Cry	
5.	Color	Blue pale		Body pink Limbs blue		Completely pink	

Score_______________

0–2: Severe asphyxia

3–4: Moderate asphyxia

5–7: No asphyxia
- Still born/macerated ____causes_______________________
  treatment at birth____
- Birth injuries____
- Congenital abnormalities________________________________
- Medication given____

Investigation Done

Date	Name of the investigation	Normal values	Patients values/result	Significance

Diagnosis (Final) ____

Drug Management

Name of the drug	Dosage and frequency	Route	Indication	Action	Contraindication	Side effect	Nursing intervention

Diet Plan

24 hours Nutritional Requirements

____

____

____

____

Nursing Care Plan

ASSESSMENT Subjective Objective	Nursing diagnosis	GOALS Short-term Long-term	Implementation	Evaluation

Summary/Conclusion

Health Education

Reference

Date of submission: **Signature of subject In-charge:**

NURSING CARE PLAN: 3

Name of the patient: _______________________ IP number: _______________

Name of the hospital: _______________________ Date of admission: _______________

Treating Doctor: _______________________

Demographic Data

Name of the patient:	Age:
Name of husband:	Husband age:
Date of first visit:	Language spoken:
Education:	Occupation
Husband education:	Husband occupation:
Family income:	Address with contact number:

Present Pregnancy Complaints

Possible problems in all trimesters of pregnancy:	
Headache/dizziness/visual disturbance/syncope/fatigue/nausea/vomiting/heart burn/shortness of breath/ abdominal pain/vaginal bleeding/vaginal discharge/constipation/hemorrhoids/ankle edema	
Bowel habits: Regular/irregular	**Skin:** Abdominal wall/groin/vulva/anal region
Lymphatic system: Enlarged gland/neck/axilla/groin/lymphangitis	**Vaginal discharge:** Red/white
Menstrual history: Age at menarche: _______________ Regular/irregular: _______________ Duration: 3 days/5 days/8 days _______________	
Past obstetric history: Anemia/neonatal death/neonatal anomaly/gestational diabetes/hyperemesis gravidarum/incompetent cervix/ polyhydramnios/postpartum depression/pregnancy-induced hypertension/preterm labor.	

History of Present Pregnancy

Gestation at first week:	EDD:
LMP:	PARA/GRAVIDA:

G_______________ A_______________ P_______________ L_______________

Family History

Type of family: Nuclear/joint family

Family Composition

Sl. No.	Name	Relationship to the patient	Age	Sex	Education	Occupation	Health status

Family Tree:

Family History of Illness
Is there any family history of: Asthma/cancer/diabetes/epilepsy/hypertension/heart disease/hepatitis/hemophilia/ stroke/tuberculosis/mental disorders/thyroid or autoimmune disorders/aged grandparent and siblings alive? If yes, what is their current state of health? If no, state the cause of death and age of death ___________________ ____ ____ ____

Past History

History of Past Pregnancy

Sl. No.	Year and month	Pregnancy events	Labor events	Mode of delivery	Puerperium	Baby status

Past Health History

Abortion history:

Pregnancy loss _______________________________________

Month and year_______________________________________

Sex of the birth: Male/female

Type of abortion: Spontaneous/induced/term/preterm/
congenital abnormalities_______________________________

Previous type of delivery: Normal/vaginal/
forceps/cesarean section

Gynecological history: Abnormal PAP, any gynecological surgery/infertility.

Past Medical history:

Hypertension/DM/heart disease/rheumatic fever/mitral valve prolapse/thrombophlebitis/asthma/allergy/thyroid disorders/gonorrhea/herpes simplex/syphilis/heart disease/rheumatic fever.

Psychological history: Abuse/neglect.

Physical examination:

- Condition of ear____________nose_____________teeth___________gums______________tonsils______________
- **Breast and nipple changes:** Tenderness/painful/warmth/presence of cyst. Nipple retraction/inverted/cracked.
- Heart sounds____
- Lungs____
- Spleen____
- Liver____
- **Skin changes:** Chloasma/linea nigra/striae (pink white). ________________
- Anal changes (hemorrhoids, edema and type) _____________________________

Antenatal examination:

General appearance:

Body built ____

Height____________________weight __________________

Vital signs: Temp____________Pulse______________Resp______________BP______________

Skin turgor: Moisture/dry

Face puffiness: Yes/No

Lips: Cyanosis/dryness

Ears: Discharge____________pain _______________

Nose: Normal/septal defect/broad/flat nose.

Abdominal examination:

- **Inspection:** Uterine size___________ shape___________ fetal movement___________ skin changes___________
- **Palpation:** Girth of the abdomen___________ fundal height___________ fundal palpation___________
  1st pelvic grip___________ 2nd pelvic grip___________ 3rd pelvic grip___________ 4th pelvic grip___________
- Auscultation FHR___________ Right side ___________ Rate per minute/rhythm___________
  location___________ position___________ left side___________ rate per minute.
  Rhythm___________ location___________ position___________

PV examination:

Cervix___________ internal OS___________ external OS___________ dilation___________ effacement___________ position___________ presentation___________ presenting part___________ adequacy of pelvis___________ discharge___________

Other examination:

- **Blood group**___________ Rh type___________ Hb%___________ BT___________ CT___________
  VDRL___________ HBs AG___________
- **Urine:** Sugar___________ albumin___________ micro___________

Present obstetrical history:

Type of delivery___________ time of onset of labor pain ___________ duration of labor ___________
medication given___________ problem after delivery___________

Newborn examination:

- Alive/still birth
- Weight of the baby___________
- Sex of the baby___________
- **Activity:** Active/dull
- **Head to toe examination:**
  - *Head:* Distribution of hair___________ condition of hair ___________ condition of scalp ___________
  - *Face*___________ presence of edema___________
  - *Ears:* Hearing capacity___________
  - *Eyes* any discharge/swelling/redness. Color of conjunctiva: Pink/pale
  - *Nose:* Any discharge/polyps
  - *Lips:* Moist or any cracks
  - *Tongue*___________
  - *Neck*___________ Neck rigidity___________
  - *Chest and thorax:* Symmetry of movement___________ breath sounds___________
  - *Extremities:* Range of motion___________

Apgar Scoring

Sl. No.	Sign	0	1–5 min	1	1–5 min	2	1–5 min
1.	Respiratory effort	Absent		Slow irregular, weak cry		Strong cry	
2.	Heart rate	Absent		Slow, less than 100		Over 100	
3.	Muscle tone	Limp		Some flexion of limb		Active movement	

Sl. No.	Sign	0	1–5 min	1	1–5 min	2	1–5 min
4.	Reflex response to flicking of foot	Absent		Facial grimace		Cry	
5.	Color	Blue pale		Body pink Limbs blue		Completely pink	

Score________________

0–2: Severe asphyxia

3–4: Moderate asphyxia

5–7: No asphyxia

- Still born/macerated ________________causes________________
  treatment at birth________________
- Birth injuries________________
- Congenital abnormalities________________
- Medication given________________

Investigation Done

Date	Name of the investigation	Normal values	Patients values/result	Significance

Diagnosis (Final) ________________

Drug Management

Name of the drug	Dosage and frequency	Route	Indication	Action	Contraindication	Side effect	Nursing intervention

Diet Plan

24 hours Nutritional Requirements

____

____

____

Nursing Care Plan

ASSESSMENT Subjective Objective	Nursing diagnosis	GOALS Short-term Long-term	Implementation	Evaluation

Summary/Conclusion

Health Education

Reference

CASE STUDY: 1

Name of the patient: _____________________________ IP number: _____________________________

Name of the hospital: _____________________________ Date of admission: _____________________________

Treating Doctor: _____________________________

Demographic Data

Name of the patient:	Age:
Name of husband:	Husband age:
Date of first visit:	Language spoken:
Education:	Occupation:
Husband education:	Husband occupation:
Family income:	Address with contact number:

Present Pregnancy Complaints

Possible problems in all trimesters of pregnancy: Headache/dizziness/visual disturbance/syncope/fatigue/nausea/vomiting/heart burn/shortness of breath/ abdominal pain/vaginal bleeding/vaginal discharge/constipation/hemorrhoids/ankle edema	
Bowel habits: Regular/irregular	**Skin:** Abdominal wall/groin/vulva/anal region
Lymphatic system: Enlarged gland/neck/axilla/groin/ lymphangitis	**Vaginal discharge:** Red/white
Menstrual history: • Age at menarche: _______________________ • Regular/irregular : _______________________ • **Duration:** 3 days/5 days/8 days: _______________________	
Past obstetric history: Anemia/neonatal death/neonatal anomaly/gestational diabetes/hyperemesis gravidarum/incompetent cervix/ polyhydramnios/postpartum depression/pregnancy-induced hypertension/preterm labor.	

History of Present Pregnancy

Gestation at first week:	EDD:
LMP:	PARA/GRAVIDA:

G_______________A_______________P_______________L_______________

Family History

Type of family: Nuclear/joint family

Family Composition

Sl. No.	Name	Relationship to the patient	Age	Sex	Education	Occupation	Health status

Family Tree

Family History of Illness

Is there any family history of: Asthma/cancer/diabetes/epilepsy/hypertension/heart disease/hepatitis/hemophilia/ stroke/tuberculosis/mental disorders/thyroid or autoimmune disorders/aged grandparent and siblings alive? If yes, what is their current state of health? If no, state the cause of death and age of death ___________________________

____

____

____

Past History

History of Past Pregnancy

Sl. No.	Year and month	Pregnancy events	Labor events	Mode of delivery	Puerperium	Baby status

Past Health History

Abortion history:	Previous type of delivery: Normal/vaginal/forceps/cesarean section
• Pregnancy loss _____________ • Month and year_____________ • **Sex of the birth:** Male/female • **Type of abortion:** Spontaneous/induced/term/preterm/ congenital abnormalities _____________	

Gynecological history: Abnormal PAP, any gynecological surgery/infertility.

Past Medical history:

Hypertension/DM/heart disease/rheumatic fever/mitral valve prolapse/thrombophlebitis/asthma/allergy/thyroid disorders/gonorrhea/herpes simplex/syphilis/heart disease/rheumatic fever

Psychological history: Abuse/neglect.

Physical examination:

- Condition of ear___________nose___________teeth___________gums___________tonsils___________
- **Breast and nipple changes:** Tenderness/painful/warmth/presence of cyst.
- Nipple retraction/inverted/cracked.
- Heart sounds___________
- Lungs___________
- Spleen___________
- Liver___________
- **Skin changes:** Chloasma/linea nigra/striae (pink white) ___________
- Anal changes (hemorrhoids, edema and type) ___________

Antenatal examination:

General appearance:

- Body built ___________
- Height___________weight ___________
- **Vital signs:** Temp___________Pulse___________Resp___________BP___________
- **Skin turgor:** Moisture/dry
- **Face puffiness:** Yes/No
- **Lips:** Cyanosis/dryness
- **Ears:** Discharge___________pain ___________
- **Nose:** Normal/septal defect/broad/flat nose.

Abdominal examination:

- **Inspection:** Uterine size___________shape___________fetal movement___________skin changes___________
- **Palpation:** Girth of the abdomen___________fundal height___________fundal palpation___________
  1st pelvic grip___________2nd pelvic grip___________
  3rd pelvic grip___________4th pelvic grip___________
- Auscultation FHR___________Right side___________Rate per minute/rhythm___________
  location___________position___________left side___________
  rate per minute. Rhythm___________location___________position___________

PV examination:

Cervix___________internal OS___________external OS___________dilation___________
effacement___________position___________presentation___________presenting part___________
adequacy of pelvis___________discharge___________

Other examination:

- **Blood group**_____________Rh type_____________Hb%_____________BT_____________
  CT_____________VDRL_____________HBs AG_____________
- **Urine:** sugar_____________albumin_____________micro_____________

Present obstetrical history:

Type of delivery_____________time of onset of labor pain _____________duration of labor _____________
medication given_____________problem after delivery_____________

Newborn examination:

- Alive/still birth
- Weight of the baby_____________
- Sex of the baby_____________
- **Activity:** Active/dull
- **Head to toe examination**
- **Head:** Distribution of hair_____________condition of hair_____________condition of scalp_____________
- **Face**_____________presence of edema_____________
- **Ears:** Hearing capacity_____________
- Eyes any discharge/swelling/redness. Color of conjunctiva: Pink/pale
- **Nose:** Any discharge/polyps
- **Lips:** Moist or any cracks
- **Tongue**_____________
- **Neck**_____________Neck rigidity_____________
- **Chest and thorax:** Symmetry of movement_____________breath sounds_____________
- **Extremities:** Range of motion_____________

Apgar Scoring

Sl. No.	Sign	0	1–5 min	1	1–5 min	2	1–5 min
1.	Respiratory effort	Absent		Slow irregular, weak cry		Strong cry	
2.	Heart rate	Absent		Slow, less than 100		Over 100	
3.	Muscle tone	Limp		Some flexion of limb		Active movement	
4.	Reflex response to flicking of foot	Absent		Facial grimace		Cry	
5.	Color	Blue pale		Body pink Limbs blue		Completely pink	

Score_____________

0–2: Severe asphyxia

3–4: Moderate asphyxia

5–7: No asphyxia

- Still born/macerated _____________causes_____________treatment at birth_____________
- Birth injuries_____________
- Congenital abnormalities_____________
- Medication given_____________

Comparison of disease condition according to book and those present in the patient.

	Theory knowledge of disease condition of patient	Present patient condition
Definition		
Related anatomy and physiology		
Etiology		
Risk factors		
Clinical manifestation		
Pathophysiology		
Investigation		
Management	Drug therapy	Nursing responsibilities
Diet		

Nursing Care Plan

ASSESSMENT Subjective Objective	Nursing diagnosis	GOALS Short-term Long-term	Implementation	Evaluation

Summary/Conclusion

Health Education

Reference

Date of submission: **Signature of subject In-charge:**

CASE STUDY: 2

Name of the patient: ________________________________ IP number: ________________________________

Name of the hospital: ________________________________ Date of admission: ________________________________

Treating Doctor: ________________________________

Demographic Data

Name of the patient:	Age:
Name of husband:	Husband age:
Date of first visit:	Language spoken:
Education:	Occupation:
Husband education:	Husband occupation:
Family income:	Address with contact number:

Present Pregnancy Complaints

Possible problems in all trimesters of pregnancy: Headache/dizziness/visual disturbance/syncope/fatigue/nausea/vomiting/heart burn/shortness of breath/abdominal pain/vaginal bleeding/vaginal discharge/constipation/hemorrhoids/ankle edema	
Bowel habits: Regular/irregular	**Skin:** Abdominal wall/groin/vulva/anal region
Lymphatic system: Enlarged gland/neck/axilla/groin/lymphangitis	**Vaginal discharge:** Red/white

Menstrual history: • Age at menarche: ________________________________ • Regular/irregular : ________________________________ • **Duration:** 3 days/5 days/8 days: ________________________________
Past obstetric history: Anemia/neonatal death/neonatal anomaly/gestational diabetes/hyperemesis gravidarum/incompetent cervix/polyhydramnios/postpartum depression/pregnancy-induced hypertension/preterm labor.

History of Present Pregnancy

Gestation at first week:	EDD:
LMP:	PARA/GRAVIDA:

G________________A________________P________________L________________

Family History

Type of family: Nuclear/joint family

Family Composition

Sl. No.	Name	Relationship to the patient	Age	Sex	Education	Occupation	Health status

Family Tree

Family History of Illness

Is there any family history of: Asthma/cancer/diabetes/epilepsy/hypertension/heart disease/hepatitis/hemophilia/stroke/tuberculosis/mental disorders/thyroid or autoimmune disorders/aged grandparent and siblings alive? If yes, what is their current state of health? If no, state the cause of death and age of death ________________________

____

____

____

Past History

History of Past Pregnancy

Sl. No.	Year and month	Pregnancy events	Labor events	Mode of delivery	Puerperium	Baby status

Past Health History

<table>
<tr><td>

Abortion history:

- Pregnancy loss _______________________________
- Month and year _______________________________
- **Sex of the birth:** Male/female
- **Type of abortion:** Spontaneous/induced/term/preterm/ congenital abnormalities _______________________________

</td><td>

Previous type of delivery: Normal/vaginal/ forceps/cesarean section

</td></tr>
</table>

Gynecological history: Abnormal PAP, any gynecological surgery/infertility.

Past Medical history:

Hypertension/DM/heart disease/rheumatic fever/mitral valve prolapse/thrombophlebitis/asthma/allergy/thyroid disorders/gonorrhea/herpes simplex/syphilis/heart disease/rheumatic fever

Psychological history: Abuse/neglect.

Physical examination:

- Condition of ear __________ nose __________ teeth __________ gums __________ tonsils __________
- **Breast and nipple changes:** Tenderness/painful/warmth/presence of cyst.
- Nipple retraction/inverted/cracked.
- Heart sounds __________
- Lungs __________
- Spleen __________
- Liver __________
- **Skin changes:** Chloasma/linea nigra/striae (pink white) __________
- Anal changes (hemorrhoids, edema and type) __________

Antenatal examination:

General appearance:

- Body built __________
- Height __________ weight __________
- **Vital signs:** Temp __________ Pulse __________ Resp __________ BP __________
- **Skin turgor:** Moisture/dry
- **Face puffiness:** Yes/No
- **Lips:** Cyanosis/dryness
- **Ears:** Discharge __________ pain __________
- **Nose:** Normal/septal defect/broad/flat nose.

Abdominal examination:

- **Inspection:** Uterine size __________ shape __________ fetal movement __________ skin changes __________
- **Palpation:** Girth of the abdomen __________ fundal height __________ fundal palpation __________
  1st pelvic grip __________ 2nd pelvic grip __________
  3rd pelvic grip __________ 4th pelvic grip __________
- Auscultation FHR __________ Right side __________ Rate per minute/rhythm __________
  location __________ position __________ left side __________
  rate per minute. Rhythm __________ location __________ position __________

PV examination:

Cervix __________ internal OS __________ external OS __________ dilation __________
effacement __________ position __________ presentation __________ presenting part __________
adequacy of pelvis __________ discharge __________

Other examination:
- **Blood group**___________Rh type___________Hb%___________BT___________
  CT___________VDRL___________HBs AG___________
- **Urine:** sugar___________albumin___________micro___________

Present obstetrical history:

Type of delivery___________time of onset of labor pain___________duration of labor___________ medication given___________problem after delivery___________

Newborn examination:

- Alive/still birth
- Weight of the baby___________
- Sex of the baby___________
- **Activity:** Active/dull
- **Head to toe examination**
- **Head:** Distribution of hair___________condition of hair___________condition of scalp___________
- **Face**___________presence of edema___________
- **Ears:** Hearing capacity___________
- Eyes any discharge/swelling/redness. Color of conjunctiva: Pink/pale
- **Nose:** Any discharge/polyps
- **Lips:** Moist or any cracks
- **Tongue**___________
- **Neck**___________Neck rigidity___________
- **Chest and thorax:** Symmetry of movement___________breath sounds___________
- **Extremities:** Range of motion___________

Apgar Scoring

Sl. No.	Sign	0	1–5 min	1	1–5 min	2	1–5 min
1.	Respiratory effort	Absent		Slow irregular, weak cry		Strong cry	
2.	Heart rate	Absent		Slow, less than 100		Over 100	
3.	Muscle tone	Limp		Some flexion of limb		Active movement	
4.	Reflex response to flicking of foot	Absent		Facial grimace		Cry	
5.	Color	Blue pale		Body pink Limbs blue		Completely pink	

Score___________

0–2: Severe asphyxia

3–4: Moderate asphyxia

5–7: No asphyxia
- Still born/macerated___________causes___________treatment at birth___________
- Birth injuries___________
- Congenital abnormalities___________
- Medication given___________

Comparison of disease condition according to book and those present in the patient.

	Theory knowledge of disease condition of patient	Present patient condition
Definition		
Related anatomy and physiology		
Etiology		
Risk factors		
Clinical manifestation		
Pathophysiology		
Investigation		
Management	Drug therapy	Nursing responsibilities
Diet		

Nursing Care Plan

ASSESSMENT Subjective Objective	Nursing diagnosis	GOALS Short-term Long-term	Implementation	Evaluation

Summary/Conclusion

Health Education

Reference

Date of submission: Signature of subject In-charge:

CASE PRESENTATION: 1

Name of the patient: _________________________________ IP number: ___________________________

Name of the hospital: ________________________________ Date of admission: ______________________

Treating Doctor: ____________________________________

Demographic Data

Name of the patient:	Age:
Name of husband:	Husband age:
Date of first visit:	Language spoken:
Education:	Occupation:
Husband education:	Husband occupation:
Family income:	Address with contact number:

Present Pregnancy Complaints

Possible problems in all trimesters of pregnancy:	
Headache/dizziness/visual disturbance/syncope/fatigue/nausea/vomiting/heart burn/shortness of breath/ abdominal pain/vaginal bleeding/vaginal discharge/constipation/hemorrhoids/ankle edema	
Bowel habits: Regular/irregular	**Skin:** Abdominal wall/groin/vulva/anal region
Lymphatic system: Enlarged gland/neck/axilla/groin/ lymphangitis	**Vaginal discharge:** Red/white

Menstrual history:
• Age at menarche: _________________________________   • Regular/irregular : _________________________________   • **Duration:** 3 days/5 days/8 days: _________________________
Past obstetric history:
Anemia/neonatal death/neonatal anomaly/gestational diabetes/hyperemesis gravidarum/incompetent cervix/ polyhydramnios/postpartum depression/pregnancy-induced hypertension/preterm labor.

History of Present Pregnancy

Gestation at first week:	EDD:
LMP:	PARA/GRAVIDA:

G________________________A________________________P________________________L________________________

Family History

Type of family: Nuclear/joint family

Family Composition

Sl. No.	Name	Relationship to the patient	Age	Sex	Education	Occupation	Health status

Family Tree

Family History of Illness

Is there any family history of: Asthma/cancer/diabetes/epilepsy/hypertension/heart disease/hepatitis/hemophilia/ stroke/tuberculosis/mental disorders/thyroid or autoimmune disorders/aged grandparent and siblings alive? If yes, what is their current state of health? If no, state the cause of death and age of death ___________________________

____

____

____

Past History

History of Past Pregnancy

Sl. No.	Year and month	Pregnancy events	Labor events	Mode of delivery	Puerperium	Baby status

Past Health History

<table>
<tr><td>

Abortion history:

- Pregnancy loss __________________________
- Month and year__________________________
- **Sex of the birth:** Male/female
- **Type of abortion:** Spontaneous/induced/term/preterm/ congenital abnormalities __________________

</td><td>

Previous type of delivery: Normal/vaginal/ forceps/cesarean section

</td></tr>
</table>

Gynecological history: Abnormal PAP, any gynecological surgery/infertility.

Past Medical history:

Hypertension/DM/heart disease/rheumatic fever/mitral valve prolapse/thrombophlebitis/asthma/allergy/thyroid disorders/gonorrhea/herpes simplex/syphilis/heart disease/rheumatic fever

Psychological history: Abuse/neglect.

Physical examination:

- Condition of ear__________nose__________teeth__________gums__________tonsils__________
- **Breast and nipple changes:** Tenderness/painful/warmth/presence of cyst.
- Nipple retraction/inverted/cracked.
- Heart sounds__________________________
- Lungs__________________________
- Spleen__________________________
- Liver__________________________
- **Skin changes:** Chloasma/linea nigra/striae (pink white) __________
- Anal changes (hemorrhoids, edema and type) __________

Antenatal examination:

General appearance:

- Body built __________________________
- Height__________weight __________
- **Vital signs:** Temp__________Pulse__________Resp__________BP__________
- **Skin turgor:** Moisture/dry
- **Face puffiness:** Yes/No
- **Lips:** Cyanosis/dryness
- **Ears:** Discharge__________pain __________
- **Nose:** Normal/septal defect/broad/flat nose.

Abdominal examination:

- **Inspection:** Uterine size__________shape__________fetal movement__________skin changes__________
- **Palpation:** Girth of the abdomen__________fundal height__________fundal palpation__________
  1st pelvic grip__________2nd pelvic grip__________
  3rd pelvic grip__________4th pelvic grip__________
- Auscultation FHR__________Right side__________Rate per minute/rhythm__________
  location__________position__________left side__________
  rate per minute. Rhythm__________location__________position__________

PV examination:

Cervix__________internal OS__________external OS__________dilation__________
effacement__________position__________presentation__________presenting part__________
adequacy of pelvis__________discharge__________

Other examination:

- **Blood group**_______________Rh type_______________Hb%_______________BT_______________
  CT_______________VDRL_______________HBs AG_______________
- **Urine:** sugar_______________albumin_______________micro_______________

Present obstetrical history:

Type of delivery_______________time of onset of labor pain _______________duration of labor _______________
medication given_______________problem after delivery_______________

Newborn examination:

- Alive/still birth
- Weight of the baby_______________
- Sex of the baby_______________
- **Activity:** Active/dull
- **Head to toe examination**
- **Head:** Distribution of hair_______________condition of hair_______________condition of scalp_______________
- **Face**_______________presence of edema_______________
- **Ears:** Hearing capacity_______________
- Eyes any discharge/swelling/redness. Color of conjunctiva: Pink/pale
- **Nose:** Any discharge/polyps
- **Lips:** Moist or any cracks
- **Tongue**_______________
- **Neck**_______________Neck rigidity_______________
- **Chest and thorax:** Symmetry of movement_______________breath sounds_______________
- **Extremities:** Range of motion_______________

Apgar Scoring

Sl. No.	Sign	0	1–5 min	1	1–5 min	2	1–5 min
1.	Respiratory effort	Absent		Slow irregular, weak cry		Strong cry	
2.	Heart rate	Absent		Slow, less than 100		Over 100	
3.	Muscle tone	Limp		Some flexion of limb		Active movement	
4.	Reflex response to flicking of foot	Absent		Facial grimace		Cry	
5.	Color	Blue pale		Body pink Limbs blue		Completely pink	

Score_______________

0–2: Severe asphyxia

3–4: Moderate asphyxia

5–7: No asphyxia

- Still born/macerated _______________causes_______________treatment at birth_______________
- Birth injuries_______________
- Congenital abnormalities_______________
- Medication given_______________

Comparison of disease condition according to book and those present in the patient.

	Theory knowledge of disease condition of patient	Present patient condition
Definition		
Related anatomy and physiology		
Etiology		
Risk factors		
Clinical manifestation		
Pathophysiology		
Investigation		
Management	Drug therapy	Nursing responsibilities
Diet		

Nursing Care Plan

ASSESSMENT Subjective Objective	Nursing diagnosis	GOALS Short-term Long-term	Implementation	Evaluation

Summary/Conclusion

Health Education

Reference

Date of submission: **Signature of subject In-charge:**

CASE PRESENTATION: 2

Name of the patient: ________________________ IP number: ________________________
Name of the hospital: ________________________ Date of admission: ________________________
Treating Doctor: ________________________

Demographic Data

Name of the patient:	Age:
Name of husband:	Husband age:
Date of first visit:	Language spoken:
Education:	Occupation:
Husband education:	Husband occupation:
Family income:	Address with contact number:

Present Pregnancy Complaints

Possible problems in all trimesters of pregnancy: Headache/dizziness/visual disturbance/syncope/fatigue/nausea/vomiting/heart burn/shortness of breath/abdominal pain/vaginal bleeding/vaginal discharge/constipation/hemorrhoids/ankle edema	
Bowel habits: Regular/irregular	**Skin:** Abdominal wall/groin/vulva/anal region
Lymphatic system: Enlarged gland/neck/axilla/groin/lymphangitis	**Vaginal discharge:** Red/white

Menstrual history: • Age at menarche: ________________________ • Regular/irregular : ________________________ • **Duration:** 3 days/5 days/8 days: ________________________
Past obstetric history: Anemia/neonatal death/neonatal anomaly/gestational diabetes/hyperemesis gravidarum/incompetent cervix/polyhydramnios/postpartum depression/pregnancy-induced hypertension/preterm labor.

History of Present Pregnancy

Gestation at first week:	EDD:
LMP:	PARA/GRAVIDA:

G________________________A________________________P________________________L________________________

Family History

Type of family: Nuclear/joint family

Family Composition

Sl. No.	Name	Relationship to the patient	Age	Sex	Education	Occupation	Health status

Family Tree

Family History of Illness
Is there any family history of: Asthma/cancer/diabetes/epilepsy/hypertension/heart disease/hepatitis/hemophilia/ stroke/tuberculosis/mental disorders/thyroid or autoimmune disorders/aged grandparent and siblings alive? If yes, what is their current state of health? If no, state the cause of death and age of death _______________________ ____ ____ ____

Past History

History of Past Pregnancy

Sl. No.	Year and month	Pregnancy events	Labor events	Mode of delivery	Puerperium	Baby status

Past Health History

<table>
<tr>
<td>

Abortion history:

- Pregnancy loss __________________________
- Month and year __________________________
- **Sex of the birth:** Male/female
- **Type of abortion:** Spontaneous/induced/term/preterm/ congenital abnormalities __________________________

</td>
<td>

Previous type of delivery: Normal/vaginal/ forceps/cesarean section

</td>
</tr>
</table>

Gynecological history: Abnormal PAP, any gynecological surgery/infertility.

Past Medical history:

Hypertension/DM/heart disease/rheumatic fever/mitral valve prolapse/thrombophlebitis/asthma/allergy/thyroid disorders/gonorrhea/herpes simplex/syphilis/heart disease/rheumatic fever

Psychological history: Abuse/neglect.

Physical examination:

- Condition of ear __________ nose __________ teeth __________ gums __________ tonsils __________
- **Breast and nipple changes:** Tenderness/painful/warmth/presence of cyst.
- Nipple retraction/inverted/cracked.
- Heart sounds __________________________
- Lungs __________________________
- Spleen __________________________
- Liver __________________________
- **Skin changes:** Chloasma/linea nigra/striae (pink white) __________________________
- Anal changes (hemorrhoids, edema and type) __________________________

Antenatal examination:

General appearance:

- Body built __________________________
- Height __________ weight __________
- **Vital signs:** Temp __________ Pulse __________ Resp __________ BP __________
- **Skin turgor:** Moisture/dry
- **Face puffiness:** Yes/No
- **Lips:** Cyanosis/dryness
- **Ears:** Discharge __________ pain __________
- **Nose:** Normal/septal defect/broad/flat nose.

Abdominal examination:

- **Inspection:** Uterine size __________ shape __________ fetal movement __________ skin changes __________
- **Palpation:** Girth of the abdomen __________ fundal height __________ fundal palpation __________
  1st pelvic grip __________ 2nd pelvic grip __________
  3rd pelvic grip __________ 4th pelvic grip __________
- Auscultation FHR __________ Right side __________ Rate per minute/rhythm __________
  location __________ position __________ left side __________
  rate per minute. Rhythm __________ location __________ position __________

PV examination:

Cervix __________ internal OS __________ external OS __________ dilation __________
effacement __________ position __________ presentation __________ presenting part __________
adequacy of pelvis __________ discharge __________

Other examination:

- **Blood group**_____________Rh type_____________Hb%_____________BT_____________
  CT_____________VDRL_____________HBs AG_____________
- **Urine:** sugar_____________albumin_____________micro_____________

Present obstetrical history:

Type of delivery_____________time of onset of labor pain _____________duration of labor _____________
medication given_____________problem after delivery_____________

Newborn examination:

- Alive/still birth
- Weight of the baby_____________
- Sex of the baby_____________
- **Activity:** Active/dull
- **Head to toe examination**
- **Head:** Distribution of hair_____________condition of hair_____________condition of scalp_____________
- **Face**_____________presence of edema_____________
- **Ears:** Hearing capacity_____________
- Eyes any discharge/swelling/redness. Color of conjunctiva: Pink/pale
- **Nose:** Any discharge/polyps
- **Lips:** Moist or any cracks
- **Tongue**_____________
- **Neck**_____________Neck rigidity_____________
- **Chest and thorax:** Symmetry of movement_____________breath sounds_____________
- **Extremities:** Range of motion_____________

Apgar Scoring

Sl. No.	Sign	0	1–5 min	1	1–5 min	2	1–5 min
1.	Respiratory effort	Absent		Slow irregular, weak cry		Strong cry	
2.	Heart rate	Absent		Slow, less than 100		Over 100	
3.	Muscle tone	Limp		Some flexion of limb		Active movement	
4.	Reflex response to flicking of foot	Absent		Facial grimace		Cry	
5.	Color	Blue pale		Body pink Limbs blue		Completely pink	

Score_____________

0–2: Severe asphyxia

3–4: Moderate asphyxia

5–7: No asphyxia

- Still born/macerated _____________causes_____________treatment at birth_____________
- Birth injuries_____________
- Congenital abnormalities_____________
- Medication given_____________

Comparison of disease condition according to book and those present in the patient.

	Theory knowledge of disease condition of patient	Present patient condition
Definition		
Related anatomy and physiology		
Etiology		
Risk factors		
Clinical manifestation		
Pathophysiology		
Investigation		
Management	Drug therapy	Nursing responsibilities
Diet		

Nursing Care Plan

ASSESSMENT Subjective Objective	Nursing diagnosis	GOALS Short-term Long-term	Implementation	Evaluation

Summary/Conclusion

Health Education

Reference

Date of submission: **Signature of subject In-charge:**

DRUG STUDY: 1

Name of the Patient: ________________________ Diagnosis: ________________________

Name of the drug	Route of administration	Dosage and frequency	Indication	Contraindication	Adverse reaction	Nursing intervention

Date of submission: **Signature of subject supervisor:**

DRUG STUDY: 2

Name of the Patient: _______________________________ Diagnosis: _______________________________

Name of the drug	Route of administration	Dosage and frequency	Indication	Contraindication	Adverse reaction	Nursing intervention

Date of submission: **Signature of subject supervisor:**

DAILY DIARY: RURAL AND URBAN COMMUNITY

DAILY DIARY IN URBAN COMMUNITY FIELD

Name of the community area: ____

Student name: ____

Year of study: ____

Date of commencement of study: _________________________ Date of completion: _________________________

Name of health center: ____

Family Identification

Name of the head of the family: ____

Address: ____

____

____

Occupation: ____

Education: _________________________________ Total income of the family: _________________________

Religion ____

Type of family: Nuclear/joint/extended

Contact no: ____

Family Composition

Sl. No.	Name of the member	Age and sex	Relationship with head of family	Education/ occupation	Health status

Family Health Status

Regular screening for health practice—Followed/not followed ____

Dental checkup—Practiced/not practiced ____

Any members of the family suffering from chronic fever. If yes write name, age, diagnosis, (if known), treatment receiving

____

____

____

Does any member have a cough for more than two weeks? ____

Does anyone have any other illness (dengue, STD, HIV)? If yes, write detail:

____

____

Is there any family history of asthma/cancer/diabetes/epilepsy/hypertension/heart disease/hepatitis/hemophilia/stroke/ tuberculosis/mental disorders/thyroid or autoimmune disorders/aged grandparent and sibling alive? If so, what is the current status of health? If not, state the cause of death and age of death.

____

____

Vital Statistics

Birth rate

Sl. No.	Date of birth	Sex	Parent's name	Remarks

Death rate

Sl. No.	Date of death	Sex	Cause of death	Name	Remarks

Marriage details

Sl. No.	Names of couple	Age	Date of marriage	Remarks

Under Five Children

Immunization status of under five children: _______________________________________

____

Specify name, age and reason for not being immunized: _________________________________

____

BCG vaccination: ____

DPT vaccination: ____

Poliomyelitis: ____

Measles vaccination: ____

Vitamin A solution: ____

Eligible Couple

Is there any eligible couple, if yes list the details:

____

Sl. No.	Name of the couple	Age	Using contraceptive method	Vasectomy	Tubal ligation	Oral contraceptive

Specify if any couple not interested to adopt family planning method (state the reason)

____

____

Using contraceptive method, if yes specify: Vasectomy/tubal ligation

____

Is any women pregnant? If yes, write the following remarks:
1. Gravida ____
2. Registered in hospital: Yes/no
3. Pregnant women receiving iron and folic acid: Yes/no
4. Women receiving tetanus toxoid____

In addition students are expected to obtain following information by observation and other methods:
1. Description of the urban community location
2. Topography
3. Climate
4. History
5. Maintain record of road to health card knowing the degree of malnutrition for under 5 (use nutritional assessment)

____

Date of survey: **Date of submission:**

Signature of subject In–charge:

DAILY DIARY IN RURAL COMMUNITY FIELD

Name of the community area: _______________________________________

Student name: _______________________________________

Year of study: _______________________________________

Date of commencement of study: _______________ Date of completion: _______________

Name of health center: _______________________________________

Family Identification

Name of the head of the family: _______________________________________

Address: _______________________________________

____

____

Occupation: _______________________________________

Education: _______________________ Total income of the family: _______________

Religion _______________________________________

Type of family: Nuclear/joint/extended

Contact no: _______________________________________

Family Composition

Sl. No.	Name of the member	Relationship with head of the family	Age	Sex	Education	Income	Health status

Housing and Sanitary Condition

- Type of house: Kutcha/pucca/semi-pucca/tiles/own/rented
- Number of rooms: _______________________________________
- Number of inhabitants: _______________________________________
- Sleeping arrangements–Provision of privacy: Yes/No
- Ventilation: Adequate/inadequate/no ventilation
- Wash room facility: Adequate/inadequate
- Living space: Adequate/inadequate
- Lighting: Electricity/gas lamp/lamplight
- Drinking water supply: Public supply/bore well/open tank
- Kitchen ventilation and light: Adequate/inadequate
- Cooking use: Fire wood/kerosene/cow dung
- Toilet type: Sanitary use–public lavatory/open air defecation

- Cloth washing facilities: Adequate/use tank water/open well
- Drainage system: Open/closed/soakage/drain/kitchen/garden/pit
- Is the sullage water being disposed hygienically: Yes/No
- Measure to control insects (flies and rodents): Present/no measure?
- System of waste disposal: Disposed hygienically, if yes/no–close to the house/separate from the house/separate from resident area (burning/burying/composing)
- Open space around the house: Yes/No
- Water stagnation: Yes/No
- Are the cattle and poultry housed hygienically? Yes/No. If yes, separate/within house.
- Is there a well or hand pump? Yes/No. If yes, is it maintained in good order? Yes/No.
- Are there any stray dogs in the vicinity? Yes/No. If yes, write approximate number of dogs__________________
- Summary: Any relevant information: ____
____

Family Health Status

Regular screening for health practice—Followed/not followed.

Dental check-up—Practiced/not practiced.

Any members of the family suffering from chronic fever, if yes, write name, age, diagnosis (if known) treatment receiving

____

Does any many member have a cough for more than two weeks? ___________________________

Does any member have skin disease (e.g., itching, patch write, age, diagnosis and treatment)? _______________

Does one have any other illness (dengue/HIV/STD)? If yes, write detail:

____

____

Is there any family history of asthma/cancer/diabetes/epilepsy/hypertension/heart disease/hepatitis/hemophilia/stroke/ tuberculosis/mental disorders/thyroid/any other? Specify ___________________________________

____

Food consumption by the family members (calculate for one day or one week) notes based on the total family income able to meet caloric requirements.

Sl. No.	Breakfast	Mid–morning	Lunch	Evening	Dinner	Total intake of carbohydrate__________ Protein_______________________________ Fat_________________________________

Note selection and preparation of food: _______________________

Any family member suffering from malnutrition? If yes, take complete nutrition assessment.

____

Is there any child under five in family who shows signs of malnutrition?

Sl. No.	Name	Age	Kwashiorkor	Marasmus	Vitamin A deficiency	Anemia	Rickets

Vital Statistics

Birth rate

Sl. No.	Date of birth	Sex	Parent's name	Remarks

Death rate

Sl. No.	Date of death	Sex	Cause of death	Name	Remarks

Marriage details

Sl. No.	Names of couple	Age	Date of marriage	Remarks

Under Five Children

Immunization status of under five children: _______________________________________

Specify name, age and reason for not being immunized: ___________________________

____

BCG vaccination: ____

DPT vaccination: ____

Poliomyelitis: ____

Measles vaccination: ____

Vitamin A solution: ____

Eligible Couple

Is there any eligible couple? If yes, list their name:

Sl. No.	Name of the couple	Age	Using contraceptive method	Vasectomy	Tubal legation	Oral contraceptives

Specify if any couple not interested to adopt family planning method (state the reason):

____

____

If any women pregnant? If yes, write the following:

1. Gravida____
2. Registered in the hospital: Yes/No
3. Pregnant women receiving iron and folic acid: Yes/No
4. Women receiving tetanus toxoid: Yes/No

Vulnerable Family Members

Sl. No.	Vulnerable family member for	Name of the member	Number	Health assessment	Problem identified
1.	Under five children				
2.	Antenatal mother				
3.	Lactating mother				
4.	School children				
5.	Adolescent				
6.	Elderly				
7.	Challenging physically and mentally				
8.	Others				

Transport and Communication Media

- Own tempo/tractor/uses private transport
- TV/Phone
- Newspaper/magazine
- Language known____
- Dietary pattern of family____
- Statement of the expenditure of the family: ____

In addition, students are expected to obtain following information by observation or other method

1. Description of the community location
2. Topography history
3. Number of school
4. No of health care agencies
5. Balwadi or ICDS center
6. Place of worship
7. Maintain record of road to health card for knowing degree of malnutrition for under 5, use nutritional assessment.

Date of survey: **Date of submission:**

Signature of subject in-charge:

HEALTH-TALK IN URBAN COMMUNITY FIELD: 1

Date and time: _______________________________ Place: _______________________________

Activities	Remarks by clinical supervisor
Preparation of area	
Group participated and number of participants	
Seating arrangement	
Self-introduction	
Introduction of topic	
Subject matter relevant/adequate	
Adequacy and coverage of content	
Method of teaching	
Clear the doubts of participants	
AV Aids used	
Interaction from the participants	
Correct use of terms and language	

Summary of health teaching topic _______________________________

____

____

____

____

____

____

____

Date of submission: **Signature of subject in-charge:**

HEALTH-TALK IN URBAN COMMUNITY FIELD: 2

Date and time: _________________________________ Place: _______________________

Activities	Remarks by clinical supervisor
Preparation of area	
Group participated and number of participants	
Seating arrangement	
Self-introduction	
Introduction of topic	
Subject matter relevant/adequate	
Adequacy and coverage of content	
Method of teaching	
Clear the doubts of participants	
AV Aids used	
Interaction from the participants	
Correct use of terms and language	

Summary of health teaching topic ____

____

____

____

____

____

____

____

____

Date of submission: **Signature of subject in-charge:**

HEALTH-TALK IN RURAL COMMUNITY FIELD: 1

Date and time: _______________________________________ Place: _______________________________

Activities	Remarks by clinical supervisor
Preparation of area	
Group participated and number of participants	
Seating arrangement	
Self-introduction	
Introduction of topic	
Subject matter relevant/adequate	
Adequacy and coverage of content	
Method of teaching	
Clear the doubts of participants	
AV Aids used	
Interaction from the participants	
Correct use of terms and language	

Summary of health teaching topic ____

____

____

____

____

____

____

____

____

Date of submission: **Signature of subject in-charge:**

HEALTH-TALK IN RURAL COMMUNITY FIELD: 2

Date and time: _________________________________ Place: _______________________

Activities	Remarks by clinical supervisor
Preparation of area	
Group participated and number of participants	
Seating arrangement	
Self-introduction	
Introduction of topic	
Subject matter relevant/adequate	
Adequacy and coverage of content	
Method of teaching	
Clear the doubts of participants	
AV Aids used	
Interaction from the participants	
Correct use of terms and language	

Summary of health teaching topic ____

____

____

____

____

____

____

____

Date of submission: **Signature of subject in-charge:**

COMMUNITY PROFILE URBAN: 1

■ FAMILY IDENTIFICATION

Name of the head of the family: ____

Address: ____

Occupation: ____

Education: _______________________________Total income of the family: _________________________

Religion ____

Type of family: Nuclear/joint/extended

Total family members: ____

Family Composition

Sl. No.	Name of the member	Relationship with head of the family	Age	Sex	Education	Income	Health status

Housing and Sanitary Condition

- Type of house: Kutcha/pucca/semi–pucca/tiles/own/rented
- Number of rooms: ____
- Number of inhabitants: ____
- Sleeping arrangements–Provision of privacy: Yes/No
- Ventilation: Adequate/inadequate/no ventilation
- Wash room facility: Adequate/inadequate
- Living space: Adequate/inadequate
- Lighting: Electricity/gas lamp/lamplight
- Drinking water supply: Public supply/bore well/open tank
- Kitchen ventilation and light: Adequate/inadequate
- Cooking use: Fire wood/kerosene/cow dung
- Toilet type: Sanitary use–public lavatory/open air defecation
- Cloth washing facilities: Adequate/use tank water/open well
- Drainage system: Open/closed/soakage/drain/kitchen/garden/pit

- Is the sullage water being disposed hygienically: Yes/No
- Measure to control insects (flies and rodents): Present/no measure?
- System of waste disposal: Disposed hygienically, if yes/no–close to the house/separate from the house/separate from resident area (burning/burying/composing)
- Open space around the house: Yes/No
- Water stagnation: Yes/No
- Are the cattle and poultry housed hygienically? Yes/No. If yes, separate/within house.
- Is there a well or hand pump? Yes/No. If yes, is it maintained in good order? Yes/No.
- Are there any stray dogs in the vicinity? Yes/No. If yes, write approximate number of dogs_______________________
- Summary: Any relevant information: ____
____

Family Health Status

Regular screening for health practice—Followed/not followed.

Dental check-up—Practiced/not practiced.

Any members of the family suffering from chronic fever, if yes, write name, age, diagnosis (if known) treatment receiving____

Does any many member have a cough for more than two weeks? _______________________

Does any member have skin disease (e.g., itching, patch write, age, diagnosis and treatment)? _______________

Does one have any other illness (dengue/HIV/STD)? If yes, write detail:_______________________
____

Is there any family history of asthma/cancer/diabetes/epilepsy/hypertension/heart disease/hepatitis/hemophilia/stroke/tuberculosis/mental disorders/thyroid/any other? Specify _______________________
____

Food consumption by the family members (calculate for one day or one week) notes based on the total family income able to meet caloric requirements.

Sl. No.	Breakfast	Mid-morning	Lunch	Evening	Dinner	Total intake of carbohydrate__________ Protein__________ Fat__________

Note selection and preparation of food: ____
Any family member suffering from malnutrition? If yes, take complete nutrition assessment._____________________
____

Is there any child under five in family who shows signs of malnutrition?

Sl. No.	Name	Age	Kwashiorkor	Marasmus	Vitamin A deficiency	Anemia	Rickets

Vital Statistics

Birth rate

Sl. No.	Date of birth	Sex	Parent's name	Remarks

Death rate

Sl. No.	Date of death	Sex	Cause of death	Name	Remarks

Marriage details

Sl. No.	Names of couple	Age	Date of marriage	Remarks

Under Five Children

Immunization status of under five children: ____

Specify name, age and reason for not being immunized: _______________________________________

____

BCG vaccination: ____

DPT vaccination: ____

Poliomyelitis: ____

Measles vaccination: ____

Vitamin A solution: ____

Eligible Couple

Is there any eligible couple? If yes, list their name:

Sl. No.	Name of the couple	Age	Using contraceptive method	Vasectomy	Tubal legation	Oral contraceptives

Specify if any couple not interested to adopt family planning method (state the reason):__________________________

____

If any women pregnant? If yes, write the following:
1. Gravida____
2. Registered in the hospital: Yes/No
3. Pregnant women receiving iron and folic acid: Yes/No
4. Women receiving tetanus toxoid: Yes/No

Vulnerable Family Members

Sl. No.	Vulnerable family member for	Name of the member	Number	Health assessment	Problem identified
1.	Under five children				
2.	Antenatal mother				
3.	Lactating mother				
4.	School children				
5.	Adolescent				
6.	Elderly				
7.	Challenging physically and mentally				
8.	Others				

Transport and Communication Media

- Own tempo/tractor/uses private transport
- TV/Phone
- Newspaper/magazine
- Language known____
- Dietary pattern of family____
- Statement of the expenditure of the family: _______________________________________

In addition, students are expected to obtain following information by observation or other method:
- Description of the community location
- Topography history
- Number of school
- No. of healthcare agencies
- Balwadi or ICDS center
- Place of worship
- Maintain record of road to health card for knowing degree of malnutrition for under 5, use nutritional assessment.

Problems Identified in the Family

1. ____
2. ____
3. ____
4. ____
5. ____

Family Nursing Care Plan

Family problem	Family nursing problem	Goals	Interventions	Methods of family–nurse contact	Resources required	Evaluation

Summary/Conclusion

Health Education

Reference

Date of survey:

Date of submission:

Signature of subject in-charge:

COMMUNITY PROFILE URBAN: 2

■ FAMILY IDENTIFICATION

Name of the head of the family: _______________________________

Address: _______________________________

Occupation: _______________________________

Education: _________________ Total income of the family: _________________

Religion _______________________________

Type of family: Nuclear/joint/extended

Total family members: _______________________________

Family Composition

Sl. No.	Name of the member	Relationship with head of the family	Age	Sex	Education	Income	Health status

Housing and Sanitary Condition

- Type of house: Kutcha/pucca/semi–pucca/tiles/own/rented
- Number of rooms: _______________________________
- Number of inhabitants: _______________________________
- Sleeping arrangements–Provision of privacy: Yes/No
- Ventilation: Adequate/inadequate/no ventilation
- Wash room facility: Adequate/inadequate
- Living space: Adequate/inadequate
- Lighting: Electricity/gas lamp/lamplight
- Drinking water supply: Public supply/bore well/open tank
- Kitchen ventilation and light: Adequate/inadequate
- Cooking use: Fire wood/kerosene/cow dung
- Toilet type: Sanitary use–public lavatory/open air defecation

- Cloth washing facilities: Adequate/use tank water/open well
- Drainage system: Open/closed/soakage/drain/kitchen/garden/pit
- Is the sullage water being disposed hygienically: Yes/No
- Measure to control insects (flies and rodents): Present/no measure?
- System of waste disposal: Disposed hygienically, if yes/no–close to the house/separate from the house/separate from resident area (burning/burying/composing)
- Open space around the house: Yes/No
- Water stagnation: Yes/No
- Are the cattle and poultry housed hygienically? Yes/No. If yes, separate/within house.
- Is there a well or hand pump? Yes/No. If yes, is it maintained in good order? Yes/No.
- Are there any stray dogs in the vicinity? Yes/No. If yes, write approximate number of dogs_____________________
- Summary: Any relevant information: ____
____

Family Health Status

Regular screening for health practice—Followed/not followed.

Dental check-up—Practiced/not practiced.

Any members of the family suffering from chronic fever, if yes, write name, age, diagnosis (if known) treatment receiving____

Does any many member have a cough for more than two weeks? _________________________________

Does any member have skin disease (e.g., itching, patch write, age, diagnosis and treatment)? _________________

Does one have any other illness (dengue/HIV/STD)? If yes, write detail:_______________________________
____

Is there any family history of asthma/cancer/diabetes/epilepsy/hypertension/heart disease/hepatitis/hemophilia/stroke/tuberculosis/mental disorders/thyroid/any other? Specify _______________________
____

Food consumption by the family members (calculate for one day or one week) notes based on the total family income able to meet caloric requirements.

Sl. No.	Breakfast	Mid-morning	Lunch	Evening	Dinner	Total intake of carbohydrate____________ Protein____________ Fat____________

Note selection and preparation of food: _______________________________________

Any family member suffering from malnutrition? If yes, take complete nutrition assessment._______________

____

Is there any child under five in family who shows signs of malnutrition?

Sl. No.	Name	Age	Kwashiorkor	Marasmus	Vitamin A deficiency	Anemia	Rickets

Vital Statistics

Birth rate

Sl. No.	Date of birth	Sex	Parent's name	Remarks

Death rate

Sl. No.	Date of death	Sex	Cause of death	Name	Remarks

Marriage details

Sl. No.	Names of couple	Age	Date of marriage	Remarks

Under Five Children

Immunization status of under five children: ____

Specify name, age and reason for not being immunized: _______________________________________

____

BCG vaccination: ____

DPT vaccination: ____

Poliomyelitis: ____

Measles vaccination: ____

Vitamin A solution: ____

Eligible Couple

Is there any eligible couple? If yes, list their name:

Sl. No.	Name of the couple	Age	Using contraceptive method	Vasectomy	Tubal legation	Oral contraceptives

Specify if any couple not interested to adopt family planning method (state the reason):___________________
____
____

If any women pregnant? If yes, write the following:
1. Gravida____
2. Registered in the hospital: Yes/No
3. Pregnant women receiving iron and folic acid: Yes/No
4. Women receiving tetanus toxoid: Yes/No

Vulnerable Family Members

Sl. No.	Vulnerable family member for	Name of the member	Number	Health assessment	Problem identified
1.	Under five children				
2.	Antenatal mother				
3.	Lactating mother				
4.	School children				
5.	Adolescent				
6.	Elderly				
7.	Challenging physically and mentally				
8.	Others				

Transport and Communication Media

- Own tempo/tractor/uses private transport
- TV/Phone
- Newspaper/magazine
- Language known____
- Dietary pattern of family____
- Statement of the expenditure of the family: ____

In addition, students are expected to obtain following information by observation or other method:
- Description of the community location
- Topography history
- Number of school
- No. of healthcare agencies
- Balwadi or ICDS center
- Place of worship
- Maintain record of road to health card for knowing degree of malnutrition for under 5, use nutritional assessment.

Problems Identified in the Family

1. ____
2. ____
3. ____
4. ____
5. ____

Family Nursing Care Plan

Family problem	Family nursing problem	Goals	Interventions	Methods of family–nurse contact	Resources required	Evaluation

Summary/Conclusion

Health Education

Reference

Date of survey: **Date of submission:**

Signature of subject in-charge:

COMMUNITY PROFILE RURAL: 1

■ FAMILY IDENTIFICATION

Name of the head of the family: _______________________________________

Address: ____

Occupation: ____

Education: ______________________________ Total income of the family: ______________________

Religion ____

Type of family: Nuclear/joint/extended

Total family members: ____

Family Composition

Sl. No.	Name of the member	Relationship with head of the family	Age	Sex	Education	Income	Health status

Housing and Sanitary Condition

- Type of house: Kutcha/pucca/semi–pucca/tiles/own/rented
- Number of rooms: ____
- Number of inhabitants: ____
- Sleeping arrangements–Provision of privacy: Yes/No
- Ventilation: Adequate/inadequate/no ventilation
- Wash room facility: Adequate/inadequate
- Living space: Adequate/inadequate
- Lighting: Electricity/gas lamp/lamplight
- Drinking water supply: Public supply/bore well/open tank
- Kitchen ventilation and light: Adequate/inadequate
- Cooking use: Fire wood/kerosene/cow dung
- Toilet type: Sanitary use–public lavatory/open air defecation

- Cloth washing facilities: Adequate/use tank water/open well
- Drainage system: Open/closed/soakage/drain/kitchen/garden/pit
- Is the sullage water being disposed hygienically: Yes/No
- Measure to control insects (flies and rodents): Present/no measure?
- System of waste disposal: Disposed hygienically, if yes/no–close to the house/separate from the house/separate from resident area (burning/burying/composing)
- Open space around the house: Yes/No
- Water stagnation: Yes/No
- Are the cattle and poultry housed hygienically? Yes/No. If yes, separate/within house.
- Is there a well or hand pump? Yes/No. If yes, is it maintained in good order? Yes/No.
- Are there any stray dogs in the vicinity? Yes/No. If yes, write approximate number of dogs__________________
- Summary: Any relevant information: __________________

____

Family Health Status

Regular screening for health practice—Followed/not followed.

Dental check-up—Practiced/not practiced.

Any members of the family suffering from chronic fever, if yes, write name, age, diagnosis (if known) treatment receiving__________________

Does any many member have a cough for more than two weeks? __________________

Does any member have skin disease (e.g., itching, patch write, age, diagnosis and treatment)? __________________

Does one have any other illness (dengue/HIV/STD)? If yes, write detail:__________________

____

Is there any family history of asthma/cancer/diabetes/epilepsy/hypertension/heart disease/hepatitis/ hemophilia/stroke/tuberculosis/mental disorders/thyroid/any other? Specify __________________

____

Food consumption by the family members (calculate for one day or one week) notes based on the total family income able to meet caloric requirements.

Sl. No.	Breakfast	Mid-morning	Lunch	Evening	Dinner	Total intake of carbohydrate__________ Protein__________ Fat__________

Note selection and preparation of food: ____
Any family member suffering from malnutrition? If yes, take complete nutrition assessment._____________________
____

Is there any child under five in family who shows signs of malnutrition?

Sl. No.	Name	Age	Kwashiorkor	Marasmus	Vitamin A deficiency	Anemia	Rickets

Vital Statistics

Birth rate

Sl. No.	Date of birth	Sex	Parent's name	Remarks

Death rate

Sl. No.	Date of death	Sex	Cause of death	Name	Remarks

Marriage details

Sl. No.	Names of couple	Age	Date of marriage	Remarks

Under Five Children

Immunization status of under five children: ____

Specify name, age and reason for not being immunized: _______________________________________

____

BCG vaccination: ____

DPT vaccination: ____

Poliomyelitis: ____

Measles vaccination: ____

Vitamin A solution: ____

Eligible Couple

Is there any eligible couple? If yes, list their name:

Sl. No.	Name of the couple	Age	Using contraceptive method	Vasectomy	Tubal legation	Oral contraceptives

Specify if any couple not interested to adopt family planning method (state the reason):__________________________

____

If any women pregnant? If yes, write the following:
1. Gravida____
2. Registered in the hospital: Yes/No
3. Pregnant women receiving iron and folic acid: Yes/No
4. Women receiving tetanus toxoid: Yes/No

Vulnerable Family Members

Sl. No.	Vulnerable family member for	Name of the member	Number	Health assessment	Problem identified
1.	Under five children				
2.	Antenatal mother				
3.	Lactating mother				
4.	School children				
5.	Adolescent				
6.	Elderly				
7.	Challenging physically and mentally				
8.	Others				

Transport and Communication Media

- Own tempo/tractor/uses private transport
- TV/Phone
- Newspaper/magazine
- Language known____
- Dietary pattern of family____
- Statement of the expenditure of the family: ____

In addition, students are expected to obtain following information by observation or other method:
- Description of the community location
- Topography history
- Number of school
- No. of healthcare agencies
- Balwadi or ICDS center
- Place of worship
- Maintain record of road to health card for knowing degree of malnutrition for under 5, use nutritional assessment.

Problems Identified in the Family

1. ____
2. ____
3. ____
4. ____
5. ____

Family Nursing Care Plan

Family problem	Family nursing problem	Goals	Interventions	Methods of family–nurse contact	Resources required	Evaluation

Summary/Conclusion

Health Education

Reference

Date of survey: **Date of submission:**

Signature of subject in-charge:

COMMUNITY PROFILE RURAL: 2

■ FAMILY IDENTIFICATION

Name of the head of the family: _______________________________

Address: ____

Occupation: ____

Education: _____________________________Total income of the family: _______________

Religion ____

Type of family: Nuclear/joint/extended

Total family members: _____________________________________

Family Composition

Sl. No.	Name of the member	Relationship with head of the family	Age	Sex	Education	Income	Health status

Housing and Sanitary Condition

- Type of house: Kutcha/pucca/semi–pucca/tiles/own/rented
- Number of rooms: _______________________________________
- Number of inhabitants: ___________________________________
- Sleeping arrangements–Provision of privacy: Yes/No
- Ventilation: Adequate/inadequate/no ventilation
- Wash room facility: Adequate/inadequate
- Living space: Adequate/inadequate
- Lighting: Electricity/gas lamp/lamplight
- Drinking water supply: Public supply/bore well/open tank
- Kitchen ventilation and light: Adequate/inadequate
- Cooking use: Fire wood/kerosene/cow dung
- Toilet type: Sanitary use–public lavatory/open air defecation

- Cloth washing facilities: Adequate/use tank water/open well
- Drainage system: Open/closed/soakage/drain/kitchen/garden/pit
- Is the sullage water being disposed hygienically: Yes/No
- Measure to control insects (flies and rodents): Present/no measure?
- System of waste disposal: Disposed hygienically, if yes/no–close to the house/separate from the house/separate from resident area (burning/burying/composing)
- Open space around the house: Yes/No
- Water stagnation: Yes/No
- Are the cattle and poultry housed hygienically? Yes/No. If yes, separate/within house.
- Is there a well or hand pump? Yes/No. If yes, is it maintained in good order? Yes/No.
- Are there any stray dogs in the vicinity? Yes/No. If yes, write approximate number of dogs_______________________
- Summary: Any relevant information: ____
  ____

Family Health Status

Regular screening for health practice—Followed/not followed.

Dental check-up—Practiced/not practiced.

Any members of the family suffering from chronic fever, if yes, write name, age, diagnosis (if known) treatment receiving____

Does any many member have a cough for more than two weeks? ___________________________

Does any member have skin disease (e.g., itching, patch write, age, diagnosis and treatment)? ___________________

Does one have any other illness (dengue/HIV/STD)? If yes, write detail:____________________________
____

Is there any family history of asthma/cancer/diabetes/epilepsy/hypertension/heart disease/hepatitis/hemophilia/stroke/tuberculosis/mental disorders/thyroid/any other? Specify ___________________________
____

Food consumption by the family members (calculate for one day or one week) notes based on the total family income able to meet caloric requirements.

Sl. No.	Breakfast	Mid-morning	Lunch	Evening	Dinner	Total intake of carbohydrate___________ Protein_______________ Fat_______________

Note selection and preparation of food: _______________________________________

Any family member suffering from malnutrition? If yes, take complete nutrition assessment._______________

____

Is there any child under five in family who shows signs of malnutrition?

Sl. No.	Name	Age	Kwashiorkor	Marasmus	Vitamin A deficiency	Anemia	Rickets

Vital Statistics

Birth rate

Sl. No.	Date of birth	Sex	Parent's name	Remarks

Death rate

Sl. No.	Date of death	Sex	Cause of death	Name	Remarks

Marriage details

Sl. No.	Names of couple	Age	Date of marriage	Remarks

Under Five Children

Immunization status of under five children: _______________________________________

Specify name, age and reason for not being immunized: _________________________________

____

BCG vaccination: ____

DPT vaccination: ____

Poliomyelitis: ____

Measles vaccination: ____

Vitamin A solution: ____

Eligible Couple

Is there any eligible couple? If yes, list their name: ________________________________

Sl. No.	Name of the couple	Age	Using contraceptive method	Vasectomy	Tubal legation	Oral contraceptives

Specify if any couple not interested to adopt family planning method (state the reason):________________________

____

If any women pregnant? If yes, write the following:
1. Gravida____
2. Registered in the hospital: Yes/No
3. Pregnant women receiving iron and folic acid: Yes/No
4. Women receiving tetanus toxoid: Yes/No

Vulnerable Family Members

Sl. No.	Vulnerable family member for	Name of the member	Number	Health assessment	Problem identified
1.	Under five children				
2.	Antenatal mother				
3.	Lactating mother				
4.	School children				
5.	Adolescent				
6.	Elderly				
7.	Challenging physically and mentally				
8.	Others				

Transport and Communication Media

- Own tempo/tractor/uses private transport
- TV/Phone
- Newspaper/magazine
- Language known____
- Dietary pattern of family____
- Statement of the expenditure of the family: ___________________________________

In addition, students are expected to obtain following information by observation or other method:
- Description of the community location
- Topography history
- Number of school
- No. of healthcare agencies
- Balwadi or ICDS center
- Place of worship
- Maintain record of road to health card for knowing degree of malnutrition for under 5, use nutritional assessment.

Problems Identified in the Family

1. ____
2. ____
3. ____
4. ____
5. ____

Family Nursing Care Plan

Family problem	Family nursing problem	Goals	Interventions	Methods of family–nurse contact	Resources required	Evaluation

Summary/Conclusion

Health Education

Reference

Date of survey: Date of submission:

Signature of subject in-charge:

GROUP PROJECT

Sl. No.	Topic	Community field urban/ rural	Number of group members	Project duration (Start date–end date)	Date of submission	Signature of teacher in-charge

APPENDICES

APPENDIX I

■ NURSES RESPONSIBILITIES FOR ADMINISTRATION OF DRUGS

Nurses are expected to know the drugs name, dosage, route, frequency, side effect, and in case of adverse effect what action should be taken, these are based on their experience, education and observation.

- Nurses should question any drug order suspected to be in error.
- Do the patient condition, symptoms warrants for receiving specific medication?
- Verify correct dosage and preparation order.
- If you found wrong medication order ask the concerned prescriber to clarify. Once nurse administer drugs without clarification and if adverse effect occurs nurses are legally accountable.
- When a doctor orders medicine dosage, rigorous verification is required because a decimal point can result in a drug error.
- Drugs should not be administered if the nurse is aware that the patient is allergic to a particular drug.
- Nurses should verify all medications they are unfamiliar with before administering them to minimize possible drug interactions.
- If a nurse is having difficulties understanding the recommended prescription order, she should confer with a senior nurse or the prescribing doctor.
- Nurses have the ability to refuse any drug that may be harmful to the patient based on their experience.

APPENDIX II

■ RIGHT OF DRUG ADMINISTRATION

Right drug	As many drugs similar form and name, clarify patient receive right drugs, patient diagnosis make sense for the right to have this medication
Right reason	As nurses administering medication for many patient and many disease condition, they are familiar with patient symptoms did the patient condition and symptoms give rationale for this medication
Right dose and route	Verify right route of medication, read the label of medication this medication for IV, IM, OR oral preparation is the correct dose being prepared and administered (check the prescribed dose against the range specified in a reliable reference) and what route medication ordered verify before administration
Right patient	Verify the identity of the patient, by checking ID band with clarification from patient and patient chart, or ask the patient to state his/her name. Confirm is this right patient to receive this medication
Right time	Depends on frequency of medication administration, administer medication according to due schedule
Right route	Is the order is for oral, IM, IV, or other route administer as per route prescribed?
Right education	Knowledge deficit will arise, before patient receive medication nurse should educate, purpose of this medication, dosage, and duration, side effect if he experience any side effect immediately report to the ward nurse
Right documentation	After administration immediately write the name of the drug, dosage, route in nurse's notes and proper signature. With date and time.
Right evaluation	Monitor the patient after administration , immediately and after 15 minutes if you suspect drug reaction frequently monitor

APPENDIX III

■ CHANGING SCHEDULE FOR IV TUBING

1.	General administration set	• The IV tubing is changed according to agency policy • With filter at least every 24 hours for central line every 72 hours
2.	Primary administration set	Change every 24 hours
3.	Intermittent administration set	Change every 24 hours
4.	Administration set used to administer parental nutrition	Change every 24 hours
5.	Administration set used to administer blood and blood product	Change after the completion of each unit or every 4 hours
6.	Anti–infective	Every 7 days
7.	Clamp off the old tubing before carefully removing if from the needle or catheter	

APPENDIX IV

■ DOCUMENTING IV THERAPY

1. Careful monitoring of IV therapy and blood transfusion administration is the prime responsibility of a nurse.
2. Patients are potential for IV therapy injury which occurs to neonates, infants, adults and elderly whom who are receiving IV medication.
3. Nurses who performing IV insertion and monitoring should document following:
   - Date and time written of starting
   - Site, type of fluid
   - Flow rate
   - Any evidence of tenderness, redness, edema, noticed and care taken.
   - Size of the catheter or needle
   - Was the name of the person who inserted? IV device is written
   - Name of the nurse who monitored
   - Date of change of set
   - Time of changing IV fluid
   - IV fluid problems and intervention

The nurse should document immediately after performing each activates, when charting is postponed until the end of the shift, important details are often forgotten. Information that charted immediately is more likely to be more accurate and complete.

APPENDIX V

■ VARIOUS SIZE OF CANNULAS WITH COLOR CODE

Yellow	24 gauze
Blue	22 gauze
Pink	20 gauze
Green	18 gauze
White	17 gauze
Ash	16 gauze
Orange	14 gauze

■ USING CATHETER AS PER AGE

Blood transfusion large bore required	20 gauze
For very small vein (pediatric)	24 gauze
1 year old	22–24 gauze
1–8 years	22–24 gauze
Older than 8 years	18–20–22 gauze
Adult patient	18–20 gauze

APPENDIX VI

■ CALCULATING RATE OF FLOW FOR CONTINUOUS INFUSION OF DRUGS

Example

Order Tagamet 200 mg to be diluted in 100 mL and infused over 20 minutes, drug available 800 mg/mL, drop factor 10 drops/min. Calculate the drop rate in drops/min.

How would you prepare the infusion fluid, use the basic want/have formula?

$200/800 \times 2$	=	0.5 mL Tagamet is required
Volume required	=	0.5 mL
Volume of D/W	=	99.5 mL
Total volume	=	100 mL

Add 0.5 mL Tagamet to 99.5 mL D/W 5%

Flow rate calculation:

$$\frac{\text{Amount of solution} \times \text{Drop factor}}{\text{Minutes to administer}} = \text{drop/min}$$

$$\frac{100 \times 10}{20} = 50 \text{ drops/min}$$

APPENDIX VII

■ BIOMEDICAL WASTE MANAGEMENT

◆ Cytotoxic waste
◆ Black bag
  – Cytotoxic waste
  – Expiry date medicine radioactive substance waste
	◆ Infectious waste
	◆ Red bag
	◆ Used and disposable plastic items like:
	  – Blood bags
	  – Infectious IV sets
	  – Infectious plastic tubing
	  – Rubber catheters
	  – Cut plastic/latex gloves
		◆ Infectious sharp waste
		◆ Blue bag
		  – Glass bottle
		  – Glass ampoules
		  – Injection vials

◆ Recyclable waste
◆ Green bag
  – Office stationary
  – Disposable paper cups
  – Tissue paper used for domestic purpose
  – Kitchen waste
	◆ Infectious waste (nonplastic)
	◆ Yellow bag
	  – Infectious dressing material like gauze, cotton, etc.
	  – Human organs, body parts and tissues
	  – Blood bags
	  – Discarded cytotoxic expired drugs
	  – Personal protective equipment, disposable gown, mask, cap
		◆ Infectious and injurious sharp waste
		◆ Puncture proof can
		  – Used needles
		  – Used scalpel blades
		  – Cannula stylet
		  – Lancets
		  – Broken glass slides cover slips

APPENDIX VIII

■ OXYGEN DELIVERY SYSTEM

Methods	Amount delivered and fraction of inspired oxygen (FiO_2)
Nasal prongs/cannula	◆ Low flow ◆ 1 L/min = 24% ◆ 2L/min = 28% ◆ 3L/min = 32% ◆ 4L/min = 36% ◆ 5L/min = 40% ◆ 6L/min = 44%
Simple mask	◆ Low flow ◆ 6–10 L/min = 35–60%
Venture mask	◆ High flow ◆ 4–10 L/min = 24–55%

Color	%	FiO_2 (L/min)
Blue	24	4
Yellow	28	4
White	31	6
Green	35	8
Pink	40	8
Orange	50	8

Catheter

Types of catheter

1. Straight single use catheter
2. Two-way Foley catheter, retention catheter
3. Three-way Foley catheter
4. Curved or coude

Available size: 5Fr, 6Fr, 8Fr, 10Fr, 12 Fr, 14 Fr, 18Fr, 20Fr, 22 Fr, 24Fr and 26 Fr.

Higher the number larger the diameter

1Fr = 0.33 mm (Fr, fraction)

Nasogastric Tube Size

Age	NG tube (Fr)
0–6 months	8–10
1 year	10
2 years	10
3 years	10–12
5 years	12
6 years	12
8 years	14
12	14–16

Classification of Bandages

Types	Names
Simple	<ul><li>Circular</li><li>Spiral</li><li>Reverse spiral</li><li>Recurrent</li><li>Figure of eight</li></ul>
Special	<ul><li>Eye</li><li>Ear</li><li>Jaw</li><li>Caplin</li><li>Shoulder spica</li><li>Thumb spica</li><li>Triangular spica</li><li>Thumb spica</li><li>Triangular sling</li></ul>
Binder	<ul><li>Scultetus binder</li><li>Abdominal binder</li><li>T. bonder</li><li>Breast binder</li></ul>

Topical Antimicrobial Agents for Burns Patient

Topical antimicrobial agents
- Silver sulfadiazine,1% water soluble cream
- Mafenide acetate 5–10% hydrophilic based solution or cream
- Silver nitrate 0.5% aqueous solution
- Silver impregnated dressing

Steps of Handwashing (WHO Recommended)

1. Wet hand with water.
2. Apply enough soap to cover all hand surface.
3. Rub hands palm to palm.
4. Right palm left over dorsum with interlaced fingers and vice versa.
5. Palm to palm with fingers interlaced.
6. Back of fingers to opposing palms with fingers interlocked.
7. Rotational rubbing of left thumb clasped in right palm and vice versa.
8. Rotational rubbing, backwards and forwards with clasped fingers of right hand in left palm and vice versa.
9. Rinse hands with water.
10. Dry thoroughly with a single use towel.
11. Use towel to turn off faucet.
12. Now your hands are safe.